Praise for *Calm Birth*

"Childbirth in America is in trouble. But that is not the major message of this wonderful book, just the opposite.… Newman offers a program called 'Calm Birth' as a potent solution. It follows the tradition of the earlier pioneers such as Dick-Read, Lamaze, and Bradley in offering practical and ground-breaking solutions to the stresses of birth, but exceeds their efforts by a wide margin. This book is essential reading for birth and other professionals who handle birth-related impacts, such as pediatricians, pre- and perinatal practitioners, childbirth educators, doulas, midwives, nurses, and others. This book is essential for expectant parents who can promote the health of their babies and prevent unnecessary negative impacts. And it's magnificent reading!!"

— William Emerson, PhD, former president, Association for Prenatal and Perinatal Psychology and Health

"Robert Bruce Newman's Calm Birth program provides couples and professionals alike a beautiful map, a method and a philosophy, to prepare for birth in a way that honors and helps them connect with their deepest innate nature and abilities. *Calm Birth* opens up a vista of hope, empowerment, inner wisdom, and confidence to trust the ability to birth naturally. Families' stories gracefully illuminate how Calm Birth ignites transformational experience in life, pregnancy, birth, and beyond. I hope you read this book."

— Wendy Anne McCarty, PhD, RN, author of *Welcoming Consciousness*

"Robert Bruce Newman's book successfully bridges ancient feminine healing wisdom and meditation to contemporary birth practices. With a broad overview of the history of birth, and deep personal knowledge of meditation, the author presents practical methods that have the power to redefine birth from a 'medical problem' to a natural human process that blesses life itself. With the possibility of safe and calm birth, bonding and trust occur easily and naturally and spread to family, community, and beyond. This book is a must for anyone interested in childbirth."

— Barbara Findeisen, MFT, former president, Association for Prenatal and Perinatal Psychology and Health

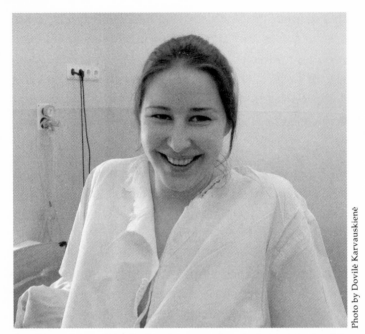

Dovile practicing Calm Birth at 8 cm—an hour before giving birth!

Calm Birth

PRENATAL MEDITATION
FOR CONSCIOUS CHILDBIRTH

REVISED EDITION

Robert Bruce Newman

Forewords by David Chamberlain, PhD,
and Sandra Bardsley, RN, FACCE, LCCE, CD

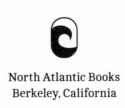

North Atlantic Books
Berkeley, California

Published by   Cover photo by Cornelius Matteo
North Atlantic Books   Cover design by Nicole Hayward
Berkeley, California   Book design by Brad Greene

Printed in the United States of America

MEDICAL DISCLAIMER: The following information is intended for general information purposes only. Individuals should always see their health care provider before administering any suggestions made in this book. Any application of the material set forth in the following pages is at the reader's discretion and is his or her sole responsibility.

Calm Birth: Prenatal Meditation for Conscious Childbirth, Revised Edition is sponsored and published by the Society for the Study of Native Arts and Sciences (dba North Atlantic Books), an educational nonprofit based in Berkeley, California, that collaborates with partners to develop cross-cultural perspectives, nurture holistic views of art, science, the humanities, and healing, and seed personal and global transformation by publishing work on the relationship of body, spirit, and nature.

North Atlantic Books' publications are available through most bookstores. For further information, visit our website at www.northatlanticbooks.com or call 800-733-3000.

Library of Congress Cataloging-in-Publication Data

Names: Newman, Robert Bruce, 1935- , author.
Title: Calm birth : prenatal meditation for conscious childbirth / Robert Bruce Newman ; foreword by David Chamberlain and Sandra Bardsley.
Description: Revised edition. | Berkeley, California : North Atlantic Books, [2016]
Identifiers: LCCN 2015051026 | ISBN 9781623170578 (paperback) ISBN 9781623170585 (ebook)
Subjects: | MESH: Natural Childbirth—methods | Meditation—methods
Classification: LCC RG661 | NLM WQ 152 | DDC 618.4/5—dc23
LC record available at http://lccn.loc.gov/2015051026

1 2 3 4 5 6 7 8 9   UNITED 21 20 19 18 17 16

Printed on recycled paper

For all those women, now and in the future,
who would love to be empowered when they give birth

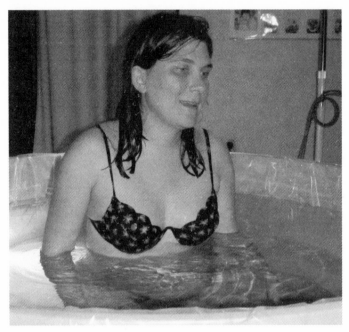

Womb Breathing: Alison in tub between contractions
a few minutes before the baby crowned.

Contents

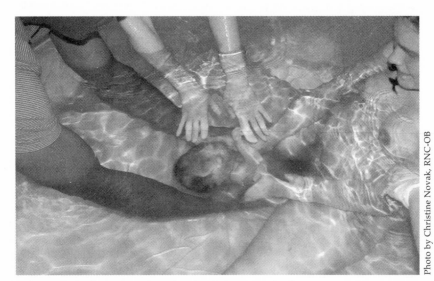

Calm Birth: Smiling Alison breathes her baby out to be born, as husband Damani (left) assists, breathing with her.

Acknowledgments

First and foremost, regarding my work in medicine and childbirth, I am deeply grateful to Shenphen Dawa Rinpoche and Chögyam Trungpa Rinpoche, two of my meditation teachers. After ten years of the study and practice of Vipashyana meditation with Chögyam Trungpa Rinpoche, I began to practice what I found to be a more complete form of Vipashyana with Shenphen Dawa Rinpoche. He transmitted the practice of vase breathing to several students of his starting in 1981. He authorized me to teach it in 1984. It was Vipashyana based on complete breathing, a more complete model of human function and potential.

At an early stage of this book's development, David Chamberlain, PhD, began to provide invaluable editorial help and guidance. David had been president of the Association for Prenatal and Perinatal Psychology and Health (APPPAH), an international association of childbirth professionals, psychologists, and researchers intent on improving childbirth practices and health. He was a widely respected author and editor. His editing of two chapters of this book, "Childbirth Meditation" and "Toward a New Era of Childbirth Education," for publication in the peer-reviewed APPPAH journal, was pivotal to the development of the book. His foreword is a testament to his understanding and support. I'm deeply grateful for his invaluable help.

But even before David's essential help with the book came Sandra Bardsley's important help in defining the Calm Birth practice. Sandra was and is a renowned nurse midwife and educator. As a midwife, Sandra had birthed hundreds of children; as an educator, she had published an important book, *Creating a Joyful Birth Experience*; and she had been one of the founders of Doulas of North America (DONA). That she wholeheartedly believes in (and has long been a teacher of) the Calm Birth practice is essential to Calm Birth. She helped define the practices, and has been a close adviser to the Calm Birth board of directors. She is vital to the program and the practices.

Sandra is currently president of APPPAH, which remains an important supporter of Calm Birth.

Other childbirth professionals who read the manuscript early on and gave helpful suggestions were Dara Knerr, CD(DONA) and Catherine Stone, CD(DONA). It's Dara's unforgettable voice that we hear on the Calm Birth audioguide, and I'm glad she was one of the Wise Women who helped make sure that the language of the book was language women wanted to speak.

I'm grateful to JoAnn Walker, RN. She was the first director of the Calm Birth program and facilitated the first interviews with women who gave birth with the Calm Birth method. Records of those interviews were the first pages of the book to be produced. JoAnn's work for the Calm Birth program is deeply appreciated. Whitney Wolf and Donna Worden were also very helpful early on in establishing the Calm Birth program, and are very much appreciated.

Anna Humphreys, CD(DONA), codirector of Calm Birth, has helped assure that the research presented in this book is up to date. Anna is committed to further updating the research in prenatal and postnatal meditation for subsequent editions of this book. I'm deeply grateful to her for her help with many aspects of the Calm Birth program. May she be ever-blessed by her devotion to childbirth health.

Foreword

by David B. Chamberlain, PhD*

A new form of childbirth preparation is spreading around the world, appropriately named Calm Birth. The innovative program is the brainchild of Robert Bruce Newman, a longtime student of Tibetan teachers, an authorized teacher of meditation, and an active participant in the new field of birth psychology (www.birthpsychology .com). Calm Birth gives women and birth professionals practical means to improve the quality of childbirth today. Like the venerable educational programs inspired by British doctor Grantly Dick-Read in 1933, by French doctor Fernand Lamaze in the 1950s, and by American doctor Robert Bradley starting in 1965, Calm Birth seeks to empower women for natural childbirth and offers ideas and practical methods for them to succeed. Like the previous programs, Calm Birth recognizes the central challenge posed by fear and pain, though its method is different, including a form of blended breathing into both the energy body and the physical body, reflecting a new vision of childbirth anatomy.

Historically, the Calm Birth program was developed by MediGrace, founded in 1991 by Robert Bruce Newman with Dr. Ted Wolff of NYU Medical Center and Dr. John Sutton and Dr. Craig Spaniol of NASA to research and develop methods of energy medicine and mind-body medicine. The first fruit of this collaboration was *Calm Healing: Medical Uses of Meditation*. Based on successful programs of the Harvard Medical School and the University of Massachusetts Medical Center, Calm Healing trainings have been presented more than sixty times in medical centers and hospitals. The pilot program for Calm Birth began

* David Chamberlain (1928–2014) was a psychologist, pioneer of prenatal psychology, and author of more than sixty publications, including *The Mind of Your Newborn Baby* (now in fourteen languages) and his latest work, *Windows to the Womb: Revealing the Conscious Baby from Conception to Birth* (2013).

in 1998 in Southern Oregon. The path created by those earlier success-ful programs opened the door for Calm Birth now being welcomed in hospitals and other birthing establishments in the United States and internationally.

Two of the Calm Birth practices have ancient roots, assuring that what is freshly presented has already stood the test of time. Calm Birth works with both physical anatomy and energy body anatomy, draw-ing on quantum physics and meditation science to access energies that are invisible but very much present.

Beginning in his strong preface, Newman provides an example of the artistic weaving of colorful motifs and original perspectives, the elevation of uncommon heroes, historical details not easy to find, succinct prose, and trustworthy analysis. Open the book anywhere and you will find this weaving of gold and silver threads.

Don't miss surprising topics like: "The Reemergence of Medicine Women," "Discovering the Potential of Childbirth," "The Wombchild's Energy Field," "Pain-Body Release," and "Awareness and Life Itself"; and the chapters of rich stories and photo illustrations of "Calm Births" (VI), "New Childbirth Medicine" (VIII), "The Evolution of Mind-Body Practice in Obstetrics" (IX), and the climactic final chapter: "Toward a New Era of Childbirth Education" (X).

When Robert and I first crossed paths in 2000, I could see that we were on a common journey. While his colleagues were mainly concentrating on empowering pregnant mothers, my colleagues were mainly busy revealing the true capabilities of prenates and newborns themselves. There was a great potential for bringing about a higher level of communication between mothers and babies than had been typical before.

From my perspective of studies in prenatal psychology, Calm Birth was arriving at an opportune time in the early years of the new millen-nium when the twentieth-century ideas about babies (and mothers) in both medicine and psychology were beginning to collapse under the weight of new evidence. An age of belief in brain matter as the sole measure of a person seemed to be giving way to a new paradigm of awareness or consciousness as the real measure of who we are.

Under the old paradigm of medicine (and childbirth education), even a full-term newborn was a creature of inadequate brain, unable to sense pain or pleasure, to have true emotion, or to think, remember, or learn anything from prenatal or perinatal experience. The luxury of that dark view permitted medical doctors to concentrate entirely on physical matters and to ignore baby awareness, psyche, or self.

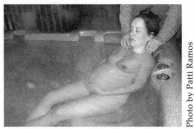

Debbie, Womb Breathing an hour before the child is born.

All three of the medical doctors who laid the foundations for childbirth education as we know it, Drs. Dick-Read, Lamaze, and Bradley, lived in that old paradigm. So did the obstetricians delivering babies, and the pediatricians who invented neonatal intensive care. Working within the narrow confines of that paradigm has presented problems for childbirth educators and even obstetrical nurses, making it professionally risky for them to become outspoken advocates for the fully sentient babies being repeatedly traumatized at hospital birth.

In the era of industrialized medicine, the refined quality of both infant and maternal awareness had been clumsily overlooked and suppressed. What began with concern for mothers in labor pain was now ending with routine use of multiple anesthetics and a cascade of other interferences—monitoring, drips, artificial rupture of membranes, administering artificial oxytocin, and dramatic surgical rescues in the form of cesareans, whether needed or not! All this has been mightily distracting to mothers and babies from doing what they might otherwise accomplish more safely and proudly together, minus all the psychic collateral damage.

Calm Birth naturally raises urgent questions about the mental and emotional quality of birth today and offers tested methods to help mothers take more responsibility for themselves and their babies. The prospect of reducing complications while increasing maternal feelings of dignity and triumph should be warming the hearts of all birth attendants.

As a psychologist, I absolutely rejoice in the idea of pregnancy as a master path for parents and look forward to the contributions of meditation science to a nobler vision of both pregnancy and childbirth.

Foreword

by Sandra Bardsley, RN, FACCE, LCCE, CD[2]

President, Association for Prenatal and Perinatal Psychology and Health (APPPAH)

The writings of Grantly Dick-Read and Frédérick Leboyer were very familiar to me when I was pregnant and delivering my own children. My births were easy and fast. Unfortunately, fairly soon after those deliveries and early in my nursing career, I saw the influence of the natural childbirth pioneers' teachings diminish as the medicalization of birth became more predominant in our culture. Women seemed to lose their innate power and internal focus. Fear became prevalent in obstetrics.

Dissatisfied, I left hospital OB nursing and went on to study traditional midwifery. Then, following a challenging automobile accident resulting in severe head and spinal cord injuries, my career path once again changed. I needed to shift the focus of my work. I wanted to stay in the area of obstetrical management, and so I decided to become a childbirth educator with Lamaze International. I also became educated as a lactation consultant and a doula trainer. Each of these paths gave me opportunities to observe my clients' responses to pregnancy, labor, birth, and early parenting. I noted that women and their support persons were thrilled with the safe births of their babies, but many women later admitted to me that they were somehow dissatisfied and depressed. I also noted that the family/partner bond was often weakened. Both the woman and her partner were not learning how to maintain their power during times of stress.

---

*Sandra Bardsley, president, Association for Prenatal and Perinatal Psychology and Health, is a respected midwife and educator, and was one of the founders of Doulas of North America (DONA). She is the author of *Creating a Joyful Birth Experience: Developing a Partnership with Your Unborn Child for Healthy Pregnancy, Labor, and Early Parenting* (New York: Simon & Schuster, 1994).

I began searching for ways to help my clients. I saw that the majority of childbirth classes of the time focused primarily on *physical* and *intellectual* preparation (what to eat, which exercises to do, what to read, whom to see for your care, and how to avoid pain using medication and interventions, etc.). The main focus in childbirth education seemed to be that of helping women move away from awareness and the feelings that were going on in their body. True, efforts were being made to include the partner in birth preparation, but the increasing use of medical technology at birth was adding confusion for them. I could find no techniques for exploring feelings during pregnancy or methods to connect and develop a partnership with the unborn baby. Very few *emotional* or *relationship* awareness techniques were available for childbirth preparation. I continued to search and experiment with teaching methods that would focus more on these two areas.

One thing I began to notice among my students was that the more often a woman focused on her unborn baby during the pregnancy, the more secure and confident she became in herself. I continued to study ways to tap into and magnify that awareness. I observed the natural desire of the woman to tune into her unborn baby to meet his or her needs. I also observed that not only was the woman striving to protect the baby, but somehow tuning into the baby was helping the woman be more relaxed and calm. I found this fascinating and wanted to learn more.

After the book *The Secret Life of the Unborn Child* by Thomas Verny, MD, was published, I became aware that the Association for Prenatal and Perinatal Psychology and Health was being organized. I became fascinated with what I read concerning this work. I joined the group studying and learning about the consciousness of the unborn baby. This organization continues to study this field of science in support of the unborn and newborn human being and society.

Following more than thirty years of research by APPPAH, science is now able to confirm for us that the baby is a conscious, sentient being, right from conception. We know that the baby is holding primal, spiritual awareness from conception throughout the pregnancy as his or her body is forming in the womb. Developing a true partnership with her unborn child becomes a great asset to the woman, because she taps into her own innate connection with inherent wisdom as she connects with the baby's spirit. In his book *Childbirth Meditation*, Robert Bruce Newman beautifully states, "When a pregnant woman turns her attention to what is innate in her, she touches upon her primal awareness, a deep basis for bonding with her wombchild. She knows that the profound awareness nature of her child and her own primal awareness nature are one."

As a result of my own growing awareness of the conscious baby, I incorporated more relaxation training into my classes. That was helpful, but superficial. There was a missing element of spiritual connection with the wombchild. During the 1990s, I had another wonderful breakthrough in my search for more ways to teach *emotional* and *relationship* awareness. I met Robert Bruce Newman and learned about Calm Birth meditation practice. I took teacher training classes with Robert and began to practice the methods of Calm Birth meditation with the pregnant women and their partners who were coming to my childbirth classes.

This life on earth is full of anxiety and stresses, big and small. How one reacts to the stresses of life is largely dependent on being able to shift one's attention from the perceived outer havoc and the chatter of one's mind, to inner peace, shifting from mind to awareness. In teaching Calm Birth meditation to pregnant women, I saw that they were able to renew their inner strength and handle stress throughout pregnancy, labor, birth, and early parenting. I also noticed that no matter what medical interventions or stresses may have occurred for the baby during labor and birth, the babies themselves appeared to be calmer and less stressed as well. The mother-baby dyad and family partnership appeared strongly bonded with Calm Birth meditation.

Calm Birth meditation became a two-way communication of great value. In preparation for the possible stress of labor and birth, the birthing woman breathes into her center and focuses on her unborn baby. This connection with primal awareness strengthens and calms her. At the same time, she is inadvertently teaching her developing baby how to also prepare for and handle possible stresses of birth and life. Through Calm Birth meditation, the baby becomes stronger and prepared psychologically for earth life, while the mother is also strengthened and relieved of stress as she reconnects with her own primal, spiritual awareness. Following the birth, breastfeeding offers another opportunity for both the woman and the baby to reconnect with their innate awareness and primordial wisdom, thus helping both to keep intact their primal connection to spirit through centering and relaxation.

I grew to love Calm Birth meditation and noted its great value for the woman giving birth, the baby, and the partner. I love how it works on a quantum physics/energy level as well as using meditation science to access energies that are invisible, but very much present. I love how it draws the woman into her own experience and power, instead of using hypnotic techniques to move away from herself and her own power. Indeed, as the woman and baby form a unified dyad, I see the Calm Birth/Calm Mother meditation practices producing a firm foundation for greater health and stability for both the woman and the child. I see these meditation practices build a stronger bond between partners, thus ensuring the baby a safer family unit in which to grow.

I truly hope you will enjoy reading this book and learning the practices of Calm Birth and Calm Mother. I have seen it repeatedly bring stability and healing to mother, baby, and partner. May you find much joy and many blessings as you learn the Calm Birth method and develop a partnership with your unborn child for healthy pregnancy, labor, and early parenting. May these blessings continue into every breath of life.

Preface

The opening up of a new paradigm is humbling and exhilarating; we were not so much wrong as partial, as if we had been seeing with a single eye. It is not more knowledge but a new knowing.

—Marilyn Ferguson[1]

How important is childbirth? How important is childbirth health? Is anything more important to human society?

Fact: The cost of childbirth in the United States is higher than anywhere else in the world, and the United States has had the worst childbirth health statistics of all industrialized nations for decades.[2] That means that the United States has had the worst infant morbidity and mortality and maternal morbidity and mortality rates of all industrialized nations for decades. Fact: The unprecedented number of malpractice lawsuits, escalating for years, has driven up the cost of birth in America.[3] Of course this is not counting the tragic likelihood that an increase of childhood diseases, and other unfortunate, newly diagnosed conditions, are results of conventional obstetric (OB) medicine. How much do we need new childbirth practice?

Marsden Wagner, MD, a scientist who has performed significant research for the World Health Organization on the extensive use of medical interventions in childbirth, has reported that the frequent overuse of inadequately evaluated medical interventions risks adverse health consequences and has escalated health care costs.[4] Not only have decades of malpractice lawsuits been driving up the cost of childbirth, they've been driving doctors out of obstetrics. Most of the older, more experienced doctors have left OB practice. The lawsuits, persistent problems of low birth weight and premature birth, cesarean deliveries at about 33 percent, and the unbearable costs of neonatal intensive care are signs of failure in maternal-infant care in the U.S. health care system. Women are forced by insurers to birth in hospitals when hospital care is the fourth leading cause of death in America.[5] How much do we need a new childbirth system?

The medical insurers have made it very difficult for women to give birth at home, even though home births are at least as safe as hospital births.[6] The insurers make it hard for women to avoid the real risks that come with the medical interventions prevalent in the hospitals. Primarily due to medical insurance regulations, currently about 99 percent of childbirths take place in hospitals, which has had a stifling effect on natural birth. Even highly motivated women who have prepared earnestly for natural childbirth are routinely overpowered in the hospital environment. The Lamaze program, the most popular natural childbirth program from the 1950s onward in the United States, currently has high epidural anesthesia rates and has high C-section rates. Cultural factors and insurance regulations have effectively channeled women into hospital birth—a relatively new form of birthing (unnatural birth) that hasn't proved to be safe or right. Despite strong national trends in the direction of alternative types of health care, in the important field of maternal-infant care, where alternatives to medical birth are needed, the Dick-Read, Lamaze, and Bradley programs have little impact today as natural birth alternatives. We deeply need new childbirth practice.

Emerging Possibilities

Are there any forces present that may bring light into the field of childbirth? The answer is definitely YES.

Medical science has been changing in ways that clearly encourages new directions for childbirth methodology. Between 1993 and 1996, three important educators described the changes needed in the health care system for the sake of national health and welfare.

Larry Dossey, MD, a widely respected medical doctor with an ability to elucidate the history and progress of medical science, published his description of "the three eras of medicine" in 1991. In his book *Meaning and Medicine,* the first of his books to become best sellers, he brought widespread attention to the development and potential

of new health care methodology. Dossey's books and other significant publications of mind-body medicine were factors effecting popular demand for an increase in availability of mind-body methods, a
demand that influenced medical and nursing schools to include alternative methods in their curricula. In 1991 the National Institutes of
Health (NIH) established the National Center for Complementary and
Alternative Medicine, expanding medical knowledge and practice.

In brief, Dr. Dossey describes Era I medicine as the scientific (or
materialistic) medicine that began developing in the late nineteenth
century and flourished through and after World War II. This is still the
prevailing methodology, intent on diagnosing, suppressing, or surgically removing physical symptoms. Era II medicine emerged in America in the late 1960s and the 1970s with groundbreaking mind-body
medicine programs at the Harvard Medical School (HMS), and then
at the University of Massachusetts Medical Center (UMMC). In both
programs, meditation was the mind-body intervention used, and it
proved to have remarkable biological and psychological benefits, especially the reduction of stress and anxiety. A factor in the development
of Era II mind-body medicine has been the increasing presence of
meditation science traditions in the West, offering authoritative methods refined through centuries of use and supported by distinguished
literature, increasingly available in English translation. The extensive
contemporary research that has developed studying the biological and
psychological benefits of meditation is remarkable in its scope. Era II
medicine implies a new model of the human body and potential.

Era III medicine is described by Dr. Dossey as "transpersonal." It
is nonlocal, universal field medicine, including such interventions as
intercessory prayer and long-distance healing, now supported by a
growing body of research. Era III medicine implies an expanded, perhaps complete model of the human body and potential. When the NIH
established the National Center for Complementary and Alternative
Medicine, it accepted the expanded model of the human body used
in such "traditional" practices as acupuncture, acupressure, and meditation, a body run by subtle but powerful energy systems affecting
the physical systems. Since 2000 there has been increasing interest

in and scientific studies of the subtle body systems, giving us fuller knowledge of human function and potential.

A second luminary of changes in the medical paradigm is Herbert Benson, MD, the HMS cardiologist who was an important early leader in the research and publication concerning meditation and mind-body medicine. Following the renowned work of Walter Cannon, MD, at HMS, which defined the fight-or-flight response and the stress response, Benson brought widespread attention to the relaxation response, an inherent meditation capability preventing people from burning out because of anxiety and stress. In 1996 Dr. Benson published his book *Timeless Healing,* based on more than thirty years of research and clinical experience in mind-body medicine at Harvard. In the book, he describes self-care as the most essential intervention for the emerging medical paradigm, and he said that the most proven mind-body self-care method is meditation. With self-care at the heart of a revolutionized health care system, said Dr. Benson, drugs and surgery would be used less, and used more appropriately. Health care costs would decline, and the standards and quality of our health care system would improve, if self-care was our primary mode of care.

A third important description of a needed and available change in health care was published in 1993 by Norman Shealy, MD, PhD, and Caroline Myss, PhD, in *The Creation of Health.* They described the needed revolution in health care to be a shift of power from doctor to patient. In the medical system that still prevails, the doctor is most often too powerful and keeps the patient in a position of weakness, which is not good for the patient's spirit and not good for the doctor. It has been widely observed that doctors and nurses in the current medical establishment carry a high degree of stress. Hospitals see that as a factor in drug and alcohol abuse by medical professionals. In a transfer of power to the patient as the primary healer, patients would be empowered with self-care training enabling them to take a vital role in their own health and healing, with mind-body methods being of central importance. Hospitals have been paying for their nurses and doctors to train in meditation for the sake of their health. Education in the use of mind-body methods is essential.

There has been no childbirth science, but we can begin to create one. It's time. We could be making significant use of the self-empowering mind-body methods now available. They are in the public domain, are remarkably well researched, and are known to medical science. The application of mind-body medicine and meditation science to prenatal care could raise the quality and standards of childbirth health care. The public must be helped to understand that important methods are available that can bring childbirth health into a new era.

Obstetrics is the area of medicine that has been most resistant to new practices of the expanded medical paradigm, practices that may have their most important application in childbirth. It's time for obstetrics to change.

Meditation is often empowering. With proper instruction and use, it has important health results for most people. The large majority of people who practice meditation properly have experienced significant biological and psychological improvements. Among the various complementary and alternative medicines (CAM) that have drawn so much interest internationally, meditation is the most researched. Meditation has become an established complement to allopathic medicine and is important to the advance of health science services. Research has demonstrated that meditation is clinically effective in both short- and long-term applications. More than twenty thousand people, including many medical professionals, have trained in the mindfulness meditation techniques offered at UMMC since 1979. Hospital mind-body medicine programs modeled after UMMC's are now available throughout North America and Europe.

Meditation's proven benefits of hormonal balancing, immune system enhancement, symptom reduction, and pain management are increasingly respected worldwide. The potential of childbirth meditation is great.

This book presents new vocabulary for a new kind of science. The glossary at the end provides deeper definitions for these terms, expanding on these ideas. Please reference it for further clarification on new or unfamiliar terms.

The Calm Birth Program

The year was 1997, approaching the monumental turn of the millennium. The place was beautiful Ashland, Oregon. I had been giving training seminars in the medical uses of meditation in Southern Oregon hospitals since 1995. With the support of the medical system, I had been instructing doctors, nurses, and patients in meditation for stress reduction and pain and anxiety management. My twenty years of study and training with Tibetan meditation teachers and with doctors had qualified me to teach what Harvard and UMMC had made famous: meditation as an important medical and health intervention.

The mindful-awareness aspect of the meditation I was trained in was similar to the practice used in the HMS and UMMC programs, but I was trained to teach the practice based on complete breathing, a different model of the human body and potential. In 1997, in Ashland, I really did have "the big A-HA!" I saw that the meditation method I was teaching, vase breathing, could be a vital childbirth practice. It would mean bringing a method with a very distinguished background into the field of childbirth.

At that time, Sandra Bardsley, RN, FACCE, LCCE, CD, one of the founders of Doulas of North America (DONA), was a close friend and associate of mine. She was also a midwife who had assisted in the birth of hundreds of children with her own hands. Sandra and other nurse friends of mine practiced the method I was trained to teach, as if it was made for childbirth preparation. Sandra, JoAnn Walker, RN, and other OB professionals who did the practice felt strongly about the potential of meditation in childbirth, and they did see vase breathing as a possibly ideal OB practice. Both Sandra and JoAnn worked with me to adapt vase breathing into Womb Breathing, modifying the practice for childbirth. As the program developed, several outstanding childbirth professionals helped make the language of the practice work for pregnant women.

The Calm Birth program was presented in Southern Oregon hospitals starting in 1998: Rogue Valley Medical Center (RVMC), Medford; Providence Medford Medical Center (PMMC); and Ashland

Community Hospital (ACH). In October 1999, Calm Birth was presented at RVMC for the combined OB/GYN departments of RVMC and PMMC. Several six-hour training seminars were presented at each of the hospitals, and a weekly class was offered at ACH. From 1999 to the present, more than one hundred teacher trainings have been held, mostly in California and Oregon hospitals on the West Coast, and in New Jersey hospitals on the East Coast, all with education credits from the California Board of Registered Nursing. Calm Birth has had the support of the Institute of Noetic Sciences. It has received grants from the Rockefeller Foundation and the Health Research Institute.

The Calm Birth method has been presented at the University of Michigan Medical School and at four world congresses of the Association for Prenatal and Perinatal Psychology and Health (APPPAH). The program has been active primarily on the West Coast, but one of the foremost Calm Birth teachers, Christine Novak, RNC-OB, was presented the March of Dimes Best for Baby award in 2009 for her work in making Calm Birth available in New Jersey hospitals. To date, probably more than twenty thousand children have been born by the Calm Birth method, in at least twelve countries. The dissemination of the MP3 files of the method internationally has spread the Calm Birth practice further than we can assess. Teacher trainings take place around the world.

Overview of the Program

There are three practices in the Calm Birth method: Practice of Opening, Womb Breathing, and Giving and Receiving. Practice of Opening is reclining progressive relaxation, using neuromuscular release and mind-body science. It allows the pregnant woman and her partner to experience remarkable access to the development of the unborn child. Womb Breathing is based on the vase breathing meditation method taught by Tibetan Vajrayana teachers. This practice offers a new vision of the body and potential of the pregnant woman. With Womb Breathing, women learn to breathe completely, to breathe energy and oxygen, to reach full potential in childbirth, profoundly enriching the child.

This practice extends natural labor pain management. The third practice, Giving and Receiving, is a treasure of ancient wisdom used to bring healing into childbirth. Variants of all three of these methods have been developed for women to use in postnatal care.

When pregnant women practice meditation, an empowering sense of safety and wholeness is generated from the inside. The Calm Birth practices were developed to give women direct ways to raise the quality of health in childbirth, whether or not medical interventions are applied. Calm Birth can be complementary medicine; it can be very beneficial if drugs, anesthesia, and surgery are used. It strengthens the immune system and helps women and infants manage the side effects of medical interventions. Meditation strengthens women psychologically. Prenatal meditation lowers OB costs and risks. It is most beneficial when used as primary care.

Given the controversial status of obstetrical practices today, and given the widespread interest in alternative health care, let us strongly consider the use of noninvasive mind-body methods in childbirth. The availability of such methods is an important chance to raise the quality of childbirth care.

—Robert Bruce Newman
Ashland, Oregon 2016

I
Background

Women have always been healers. Cultural myths from around the world describe a time when only women knew the secrets of life and death, and therefore they alone could practice the magical art of healing.... The emergence of women whose consciousness blends with the ancient themes of healing is the single most promising event in health care...

—Jeanne Achterberg [7]

Repression of the Natural Genius of Women

In 1998 I read Jeanne Achterberg's highly respected book, *Imagery in Healing,* a well-researched classic of mind-body medicine. In it is a concise chapter called "Imagery and the History of Medicine." I read it and was deeply shocked. I had of course heard of terrible witch hunts long ago, but I had no idea how far-reaching the murder was, how horrifyingly vast the scale of the killing, in Europe and America. At the heart of it were men ready and able to kill women, to burn them publicly, with full church support, because the women were suspected of practicing medicine, which the men wanted complete control of. Achterberg writes:

> In the midst of the atmosphere of change brought about by the issuance of the official mandates determining who should administer to the sick ... one of the saddest events in the history of women and healing began: the great witch hunt. It was inordinately successful in eliminating women's influence on the healing arts up to the present day. In fact, it was inordinately successful

in eliminating women, period. Estimates are that anywhere from a few hundred thousand to nine million women were murdered between the years 1500 and 1650, many of them for the suspicioned practice of medicine.[8]

Imagine the violent insanity of such a species. It's able to tragically murder its women healers, massively, and survive. And let's remember all the wrongly accused women who burned. It was the long ending to the ages of the circle of women.

Throughout the ages, childbirth took place among women. Childbirth everywhere was in the hands of experienced midwives and other women, family and friends. There were women of wisdom who were called upon as needed. Spiritual knowledge of childbirth was transmitted through the ages in the Wise Woman tradition. Childbirth was in the right hands. Most women had some knowledge of midwifery and the healing arts.

Then, in the sixteenth and seventeenth centuries, came the Church of the Inquisition and the widespread execution of women of the families of Europe and America. It was the ultimate witch hunt, through more than two centuries. Women who practiced healing arts and midwifery were primary targets. Women traditionally not only had the responsibility and knowledge to take care of childbirth; they also had profound and widely respected medicine traditions, and they took care of the dying. Coming out of the Middle Ages into the "Renaissance," Europe was ravaged and impoverished by war and disease. The competition for resources was severe. Only men were allowed to study medicine. If a woman showed a gift for healing, she was usually damned by the Church as having obtained power through alliance with the devil; to male doctors it usually meant that she was practicing medicine without a license, something they controlled.

And so it proceeded for more than two hundred years, with twisted Church authority suspecting women in general of readiness for pacts with "the devil," that the persecution, torture, and murder of women sent waves of terror through the women of Europe and then America. Some men were perfect accomplices, especially doctors and other professionals organizing to protect their authority. They gave backbone and fire to the holocaust. Burning was the favored means of murder. Alliance of Church and state conspired to create, in Achterberg's words, "the shocking nightmare, the foulest crime, and deepest sense of shame of Western civilization, the blackout of everything that *homo sapiens*, the reasoning man, has ever upheld."[9]

The institutionalization of the trials, tortures, and executions was well documented. It was the lowest level of aggressive, competitive greed in nations short of money and weak in industry, based on the power of the Church to accuse and to sanction killing. Man against woman. Achterberg continues:

> The charge of witchcraft became the single most effective means of controlling the monopoly of the healing professions...[10] Midwifery and folk healing—risky occupations in which the practitioner was doubly damned—were alternatives to starvation.[11]

Sometimes women were allowed to practice midwifery, but the profession had a bad reputation and was dangerous. Midwives were often fined, imprisoned, or killed if the outcome of their work was considered a failure, i.e., a stillborn or deformed child. And so women were hideously persecuted and punished, with their terrified families watching, for naturally being the healers and midwives the species needed.

The Reemergence of Medicine Women

The term *Homo sapiens* means wisdom man and wisdom woman. In a dark period of Western civilization, the natural gifts of the wisdom woman were repressed with torture and murder. Woman's work as a healer and her inner access to important knowledge of childbirth, vital human resources, were almost obliterated. But the species silently survived. Male doctors continued to organize and professionalize their business, taking over childbirth.

Coming into the eighteenth century, the persecution of woman the healer and midwife slowly stopped. But for two centuries after the hellish repression, natural childbirth options were generally not available to women due to possible prosecution. Licensed doctors, always men, were most often called upon to deliver children.

Coming into the twentieth century, obstetrics and gynecology were predominantly male professions that applied the interventions of medical science more and more, forming a tradition of unnatural childbirth. Today there are increasing numbers of women OB/GYNs in our medical system, but women in general in our culture are still not instructed about natural birth options.

Natural childbirth programs began to develop in the West in the twentieth century by way of two European doctors, Grantly Dick-Read of England and Fernand Lamaze of France. They both stirred interest in normal childbirth in Europe and America. Late in the twentieth century, when it was clear that the quality of human health was at risk from the uncontrolled use of anesthesia, surgery, and strong drugs in childbirth, the natural childbirth programs of Dick-Read, Lamaze, and Robert Bradley drew the attention of many women. In those childbirth education programs, women found that instruction in natural childbirth capability and prenatal care was essential for making conscious decisions affecting health in childbirth.

Toward the end of the twentieth century, teachers from revered meditation traditions coming into the West became an increasing resource of wisdom and methods. This resource has been slowly brought into childbirth and is helping women discover remarkable innate capability, helping them find healing in the childbirth process. These methods from ancient wisdom, and new methods from mind-body medicine, are inspiring new childbirth methodology. They give women the option to make childbirth a process of personal empowerment and at the same time protect human evolution.

The Wise Woman tradition is emerging anew. One way it emerges is when it comes from within as women practice meditation and healing methods in preparation for childbirth, sitting into their inherent wisdom.

New Childbirth Anatomy and Potential

It started late in the twentieth century, and now early in the twenty-first century a force of history is expanding the vision of childbirth anatomy and the potential of normal birth.

In meditation science traditions available throughout the West, people learn to breathe vital energy for greater function. In Zen Buddhist meditation, people breathe down into the *hara*, the vital navel center, for optimal function.

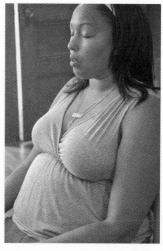

Photo by Judith Halek

In Vajrayana Buddhist meditation, people learn to breathe energy down into the Life Vase in the navel center. In T'ai Chi, people sink *chi* into the *tan tien*, in the navel, for energy and realization. Widespread interest in the work of Carlos Castaneda finds an ancient Western lineage in which women are known to be able to see and use energy and to use their wombs to process knowledge directly for evolution.

We are made to breathe completely. Traditional wisdom knows how to breathe vital energy for human development. It's a well-known meditation practice. The ability to breathe energy into the navel center in the energy body is an important human resource that should be indicated to women for childbirth.

As more and more women practice meditation, they're taking superior prenatal care when they become pregnant and practice. Some women practice breathing vital energy into the navel center of their energy systems to benefit the birth. For such women, pregnancy has become an empowering master path. If energy breathing meditation is applied as a primary prenatal care method, conception to delivery can be a path on which women empower themselves to reduce or eliminate risks and side effects of medical interventions and to increase maternal and infant health.

II
Prenatal Meditation

Meditation is not just a practice, it is a way of life. Initially that way of life is learned through formal practice, just as we learn to play a musical instrument. Some people will choose to continue [meditation] practice periods and others won't, but both will have shifted the paradigm through which they relate to the world.

—Joan and Miroslav Borysenko[12]

Both the words "medicine" and "meditation" come from the Latin word *mederi,* which means "to cure." Medicine refers to methods for the curing of symptoms of disease. Meditation refers to methods that go deeper, to shift and improve human function. Meditation is a consciousness discipline that enables people to experience greater levels of awareness and intelligence and greater levels of health, normally blocked by the mind in its undisciplined activity. Meditation science is based in profound traditions and has extensive knowledge of short-term and long-term benefits of its methods. Contemporary science has defined meditation as having five main characteristics: specific method; muscle relaxation; logic relaxation (i.e., to suspend analyzing, judging, and expectation); self-induced state; and control of attention.[13] Prenatal meditation is the application of meditation methods for maternal and infant health, for prenatal child development, and for labor and delivery.

With the progressive increase of the presence of meditation lineages and traditionally trained meditation teachers in the West in the past fifty years, and with meditation now widely accepted as a valuable health aid, hundreds of thousands of women who practice meditation have experienced benefits during pregnancy and labor. Some women who have no prior experience seek meditation and yoga methods to benefit their pregnancies.

The Increasing Presence of Meditation in the West

The presence of meditation in Western life in the post–Cold War era has become ubiquitous. As Michael Murphy and Steven Donovan state in their book *The Physical and Psychological Effects of Meditation:*

> Meditation ... is fast appearing in unexpected places throughout modern American culture. Secretaries are doing it as part of their daily noon yoga classes. Preadolescent teenagers dropped off at the YMCA by their mothers on a Saturday morning are learning it as part of their karate training. Truck drivers and housewives in the Stress Reduction Program at the University of Massachusetts Medical Center are practicing a combination of Hindu yoga and Buddhist insight meditation to control hypertension [and manage pain]. Star athletes prepare themselves for a demanding basketball game with centering techniques learned in Zen.[14]

The increasing use of meditation in different aspects of medicine has been obvious because of media attention and public interest. Since the start of the landmark research at the Harvard Medical School in the 1960s, and particularly since the advent of the medicine/meditation program at the University of Massachusetts Medical Center (UMMC) starting in 1979, meditation has been widely researched and used increasingly in medical and psychological applications. The many thousands of research abstracts compiled by Murphy and Donovan (in 1999 and again in 2010) enable us to appreciate the extensive research on the benefits of meditation, and to evaluate the benefits important for prenatal and postnatal care.

Benefits of Childbirth Meditation: Evidence-Based Medicine

Evidence-based medicine (EBM) seeks to assess the strength of evidence of the risks and benefits of treatments (including lack of medical treatment) and diagnostic tests. This helps clinicians consider whether or not any treatment will do more good than harm.

The risks of the use of anesthesia, drugs, and surgery in pregnancy and childbirth are well documented.[15] Malpractice lawsuits resulting from such procedures are remarkably extensive.[16]

Prevalent OB practice also includes risks that such medical practices may result in any of a variety of childhood health problems and diseases.[17]

The evidence cites further risk in that the prevalent OB procedures take place in hospitals, and the American Medical Association has been telling us for decades that hospital care is the fourth most frequent cause of death in America.

Because no medical treatment may be the best treatment for most childbirths, with respect to risk and health, and because "first, do no harm" is the first principle of medicine, it is best to safeguard maternal and infant health in childbirth by offering women healthy, evidence-based alternatives to medical birth.

The benefits of meditation as a childbirth intervention are supported by more than eighty thousand research papers and books published on the biological and psychological benefits.

Prenatal meditation is evidence-based medicine because meditation itself is proved to reduce or avoid medical risks, and has proven biological and psychological benefits.

The following is a brief overview of the psychological and physiological benefits of meditation that may be imparted to a wombchild through the pregnant woman's bloodstream and through sympathetic resonance. The same benefits, in general, may be imparted to the child after birth with postnatal meditation, through lactation and breastfeeding, and through sympathetic resonance. At all times, childbirth meditation benefits are dual, inseparably benefiting the woman

17

and the child. In addition, in a larger sense, childbirth meditation can be seen to benefit the family and society in general.

Biological Benefits

This subject has become vast, but with respect to directly affecting the quality of childbirth, the focus will be primarily on three concerns: hormonal balance, immune system enhancement, and pain management.

Our era has been called the Age of Anxiety. It's been well proved that anxiety and the stress it causes are key factors in the decline of health, and are significant factors in most disease pathology, physical and mental. As extensive research has shown, meditation is a noninvasive antidote to biological and psychological problems caused by anxiety and stress.

In brief, anxiety causes an overproduction of the hormones adrenaline and cortisol, which suppress important biological functions in order to shift energy into muscle systems for a "fight or flight" reaction, based on old instinctive tendencies. Anxiety suppresses immune system function primarily through elevated levels of cortisol in the bloodstream. Anxiety during pregnancy today just might be the most challenging it's ever been for women in general.

The widespread chemical treatment of anxiety has resulted in additional biological and psychological problems. If a woman is pregnant, the treatment of anxiety with mood-modulating chemicals can result in birth defects or other long-term health problems for the child.[18]

However, meditation, the relaxation response, is a powerful inherent human system that spontaneously counteracts stress, usually when people adjust their breathing and calm down.

Self-calming meditation has been shown to directly reduce adrenaline and cortisol secretion, naturally restoring hormonal balance in general and normalizing immune system function. In addition, meditation produces elevated levels of the major hormones melatonin and DHEA, as well as serotonin, and endorphins, powerful pain-relieving, pleasure-causing agents secreted by the nervous system.

Melatonin

The fact that meditation produces elevated levels of melatonin, the hormone secreted by the pineal gland located near the center of the brain, was first disclosed by research conducted at the University of Massachusetts Medical Center in 1995. The pineal gland has drawn the attention of human insight for a long time. It is sometimes called "the third eye." In sacred literature more than 2,500 years old, the Vedas of India described the pineal gland in the context of the human energy systems:

> The [pineal] gland was portrayed as one of the seven chakras, or centers of vital energy, which are arranged along the central axis of the body. The pineal gland was thought to be the supreme or crown chakra ... the ultimate center of spiritual force.[19]

In the seventeenth century, Descartes, in his famous *Treatise of Man*, called the pineal gland the seat of the human psyche, the principal location of self-awareness. Current worldwide interest in melatonin, evident in the presence of hundreds of research papers and books on the hormone, is focused on its biological benefits, particularly concerning the remarkable effects of melatonin on the human immune system. Melatonin may be the most potent and versatile antioxidant. It directly stimulates interleukin-2 activity that in turn stimulates the increase of all the various cells of the immune system, in a global optimization of immune function. Melatonin directly restores and increases T-helper cell production in bone marrow.

In stress-inducing times, which tend to cause detrimental hormonal imbalances, elevated levels of melatonin, intentionally produced by pregnant women in meditation, indicate effective prenatal care.

Melatonin is renowned as a sleep aid. Especially when produced naturally to elevated levels, it can make deep sleep and rest possible even in challenging situations. Melatonin is known to have a calming effect, bringing contentment and improved mood.[20] In our times, a pregnant woman's self-induced meditation calm may be a womb-child's greatest need.

To summarize, the natural production of elevated levels of melatonin in meditation, conveyed to the child prenatally through the woman's bloodstream and postnatally through breastfeeding, brings remarkable immune enhancement, calming, and other health benefits. Also, with prenatal meditation the woman's elevated melatonin levels are a probable intelligence enhancement factor for the child. This subject warrants extensive research.

DHEA

Increased levels of DHEA (dehydroepiandrosterone), a life-enhancing hormone, were one of the first biological benefits of meditation to be observed. DHEA is produced in the adrenal glands, just above the kidneys.

Like melatonin, DHEA has a variety of health-increasing benefits. It is an immunity enhancement agent that has been proved to be beneficial in the prevention and treatment of cancer, cardiovascular disease, diabetes, lupus, and other disorders. DHEA stimulates the production of monocytes (T cells and B cells), potent immunity-enhancing biochemicals that cause the production of other immune system agents. T cells (white blood cells produced in the bone marrow) produce two powerful immune system agents: interleukin-2 and gamma interferon, intelligent defense agents that help maintain health.

DHEA is beneficial for the bones, muscles, blood pressure, vision, and hearing. It is the substance from which the male and female hormones are developed. It contributes to vitality and youthfulness. DHEA is a mood elevator that makes people feel and look better. It enhances brain biochemistry and growth. Anxiety and stress lower DHEA levels in the bloodstream; meditation elevates DHEA levels.

Thus meditation during pregnancy, in offering potentially ideal hormonal function, generates elevated levels of vivifying DHEA in the woman's bloodstream, which benefits the wombchild. If the mother keeps meditating after giving birth, the child can receive the DHEA enrichment through lactation and breastfeeding.

Serotonin

Another important hormone produced in elevated amounts by meditation with important implications for childbirth is serotonin. It is a natural substance the body uses to make melatonin. Serotonin is a neurotransmitter produced in the brain and gut that has a calming effect, associated with contentment. It also regulates blood vessel elasticity, helps repair muscle tissue damage, and is generally beneficial in healing. It is conveyed from woman to child with the other meditation hormones.

Because of a diagnosis of stress-related serotonin deficiency, some women have been prescribed tranquilizers, with disastrous consequences. Women who meditate will tend to have less or no need for mood-altering drugs.

Endorphins

Meditation is also known to produce endorphins, peptides secreted throughout the nervous system that have a very strong pain-relieving and pleasure-inducing effect, similar to that of morphine. In the words of Deepak Chopra:

> Thus the brain [and nervous system in general] produces narcotics up to 200 times stronger than anything you can buy... with the added boon that our own pain-killers are non-addictive. Morphine and endorphins both block pain by filling a certain receptor on the neuron and preventing other chemicals that carry the message of pain from coming in, without which there can be no sensation of pain, no matter how much physical provocation is present.[21]

Michel Odent observes that the longer and more challenging the labor, the higher the level of endorphins.[22] With respect to prenatal meditation, it is probable that the more time that is devoted to the practice, the higher the level of endorphins during labor and at birth. Thus women who meditate for childbirth are likely to have optimal endorphin levels supporting the potential of natural childbirth. If medical or surgical procedures are used, the elevated endorphin levels help reduce discomfort and pain.

Endorphin production is important to a woman for avoiding risks of medical interventions and in gaining confidence in her natural abilities in childbirth. Dr. Candace Pert writes about her third childbirth:

> ... my magic bullet had been breathing, which is a surefire, proven strategy for releasing endorphins and quelling pain. Obviously, this is what previous generations of women, in the days before IV drips and synthetic painkillers, had relied on. Both they and their babies must have been better off for the experience, as I certainly felt myself to be.[23]

Meditation and Pain Management

Another important meditation benefit is increased tolerance of pain based on psychological factors. Research conducted at the UMMC[24] has demonstrated reductions in the following: present moment pain, negative body image, inhibition of activity (movement limitation), psychological disturbance, anxiety and depression, and the need for pain-related drugs. All of the above were reduced or eliminated through the UMMC meditation program. It works with a simple but profound recognition.

With the mindfulness meditation used in the program, people learn to recognize the difference between mind and awareness. They are instructed to sit and to shift attention from mind to awareness, to experience a vital change of function. As people learn to expose mind to awareness, they learn to not react to their mind. They learn to see how the mind tends to dwell on anxiety and fear and burns up energy, exhausting them and limiting their ability. With mindfulness meditation, they learn that they're capable of staying in the present moment by not reacting to mind, even while experiencing high levels of pain. They see that their mind likes to avoid being present by making a big deal about the pain. They see that for good and right reasons they want to stay in open awareness and avoid mind and its suffering.

People practicing mindfulness meditation see that they can develop fearlessness and gain energy by staying with pain sensations, avoiding letting their mind agonize and waste energy reserves. They see that they have a choice to prevent their distress and build courage and inner strength in the process.

These results point out how meditation has important potential application in labor pain management, to avoid unnecessary anguish, to maintain clarity, and perhaps to avoid the use of risky medical interventions. Staying with present moment pain naturally releases endorphins, increasing the ability to stay present. The more one is willing to accept labor contractions with meditation, the higher the endorphin levels and the greater the experience of birth.

Other Psychological Benefits of Meditation

Murphy and Donovan describe extensive research in the following benefits of meditation:

» Perceptual ability
» Reaction time and physical motor skill
» Field independence
» Concentration and intelligence
» Empathy
» Creativity
» Self-actualization

It is observed, in brief, that various meditation schools offer methods to cultivate clarity, psychological flexibility, efficiency, and a broadened range of functions. This is seen in the meditation results observed in the compiled research abstracts in the Murphy and Donovan work.[25]

The above cognitive benefits produced by meditation in a pregnant woman encourage the wombchild, through sympathetic resonance, to develop vital cognitive qualities. Future research will hopefully seek to observe and compare traits developed in children exposed to prenatal meditation with traits developed in children without that exposure.

Prenatal Meditation Research

In their important 2008 study, Cassandra Vieten and John Astin concluded what common sense and countless thousands of women who
meditated during pregnancy have indicated: meditation significantly
reduces prenatal anxiety and stress. "Experts suggest that the practice of meditation by the mother can reduce high levels of neurolog-
ical and endocrine [stress] chemicals that could be detrimental to
the newborn."[26]

Several other studies of the use of prenatal and perinatal mindfulness meditation reveal further psychological benefits. In "Mindfulness
Approaches to Childbirth and Parenting," by Hughes, Williams, Bar-
dacke, and colleagues,[27] mindfulness meditation is seen to be increasingly used as a way of managing pain, reducing stress and anxiety,
reducing the risk of perinatal depression, and increasing "availability" of attention for the infant. The authors also describe the effects
of family meditation during the perinatal period. A study in 2009 by
the Vivekananda Yoga Research Foundation called "Meditation Benefits for Pregnancy" found that a daily practice of meditation and yoga
during pregnancy seems to improve birth weight, reduce premature
births, and lessen overall medical complications for newborns.[28]

Two recent studies from Thailand are significant, particularly for
childbirth in the United States, because of the great concern about
preterm birth, a primary factor in the high infant morbidity and mortality rates in the United States. The major Thai hospital study on the
prevention of preterm birth through the intervention of meditation is
important. The study concludes that meditation is a promising technique
for reducing the incidence of preterm birth. That research continues.[29]

Another recent hospital study in Thailand, "Incorporating Buddhist
Clear Clean Mind Meditation into Natural Childbirth Practices," concludes: "Clear Clean Meditation should be encouraged during natural
childbirth, through labor and delivery, in other hospitals in Thailand."[30]

A significant clinical trial in prenatal meditation was conducted
at the Queen Elizabeth Hospital in Hong Kong in 2014[31] under the
direction of K. P. Chan, MD. Sixty-four pregnant Chinese women were

trained in a six-week prenatal mindfulness meditation course with one session a week, compared with a control group of fifty-nine healthy pregnant women who did not meditate. This clinical trial was performed to explore the effects of prenatal meditation on infant behaviors. Cortisol levels were checked via umbilical cord blood samples and then via saliva samples at six weeks and at five months. The conclusion of the trial was that the children of the meditation intervention group had better health and were less stressed than the children of the control group. They had good responses and better temperament at five months. Because of the impressive biological evidence, the researchers recommended that pregnancy care providers should provide prenatal meditation to pregnant women.

Other observed benefits of meditation with significant implications for childbirth are as follows: Astin[32] concluded that mindfulness meditation may be an important coping strategy for transforming the ways in which we respond to life events. Benson noted cesarean section surgery was reduced by 56 percent and epidural anesthesia use was reduced by 85 percent among meditators.[33]

Altogether, increased pain management skills, increased levels of endorphins, melatonin, DHEA, and other beneficial hormones, all the result of meditation, should be important incentives for women who want to reduce the risks and side effects of medical interventions and practice a better kind of childbirth than has been prevalent.

A pregnant woman's meditation always has dual benefits. The woman communicates psychologically and energetically, influencing the child to produce healthful neurohormones and neurotransmitters. She also sends hormonal benefits through her bloodstream into the child. If anesthesia is used, and/or drugs, some of which are toxic,[34] prenatal meditation can counter side effects of the medicine in them both. Though research in the benefits of meditation is vast, there has been too little research into the benefits of prenatal meditation. Given the controversial status of medical childbirth throughout the industrialized nations, research in prenatal, perinatal, and postnatal meditation should be a priority.

Discovering the Potential of Childbirth

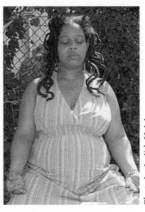

Photo by Judith Halek

Pregnant women practicing prenatal meditation experience greater function, biologically and psychologically. The practice can give the women a new sense of body and capability. Meditation gives them a vital active involvement in the pregnancy. They can experience the awareness and potential of the child in their womb as they enrich the child and themselves. Among all the variety of women who will benefit from prenatal meditation, they will each realize more of their own biological and psychological potential, and each will uniquely sense the great enrichment potential of childbirth preparation.

III
Childbirth in the Human Energy System

The study of the human energy system and the power of our own natures is the study of the dynamics of creation itself and of the vital part we play as participants in the process of the continuation and maintenance of life.

—Caroline Myss[35]

The "New" Human Body

Barbara Brennan, a NASA research scientist, published her important studies of the human energy field (HEF) and the universal energy field (UEF) in 1987, presenting a dynamic union of the physical human body and its energy body, extending beyond its skin. "The Human Energy Field ... can be described as a luminous body that surrounds and interpenetrates the physical body..."[36] Brennan goes on to describe the human energy body from her own scientific observation and insight, and it confirms what traditional sciences have long said about the human body: The physical body is governed by subtle energy power centers and channel systems that run the physical systems.

In his book *Energy Medicine*, James Oschman published his revolutionary research into the nature of the human body, using scientific advances to see further into the dynamics of mind-body function:

Much of the seeming magic and mystery surrounding vibrational medicines is being revealed as the same mystery that has always been associated with the invisible yet palpable forces of nature. Many of the subtleties arising in the clinical context are none other than the subtleties of human structure and patterns of energy in interaction. As new research reveals the basis for these subtleties, we obtain a much clearer picture of the human body in health and disease. The medical and chemical-pharmacological models that have served us well in the past are not being replaced, but are being viewed within a more complete multidimensional perspective. "Subtle energies" and "dynamic energy systems" are neither supernatural nor do they require a revision of physics. They go to the foundation of life.[37]

Claude Swanson's extensive study of the human body[38] is based on the expanding field of research into the physics of the energy body, evidence of the nature of the energy meridians and power centers. As research reveals more and more modes of energy body interaction with the physical body, Swanson senses that the potential of the human body is increasing.

Dr. Oschman says that we're not replacing the medical model of the human body, but we're viewing it with "a more complete multi-dimensional perspective."[39] Advances in science have given us a vision of the human body that sees powerful subtle energies and dynamic energy systems. If we apply this model of the energy body/physical body to the pregnant woman preparing for childbirth, we should teach women a more complete vision of what they are and can be. The more we see what we are, the more we see we may be unlimited. A woman's recognition and use of her energy system can bring a sense of new body to the most essential human event.

The Wombchild's Energy Field

Frédérick Leboyer observed the meditative energy nature of the child in the womb. Sensing what he calls the slowness of the time of the unborn child, Leboyer says softly:

Near-darkness ... silence ...

A profound peace steals over everything, almost unnoticed.

People don't raise their voices in church.

On the contrary, instinctively, they lower them.

And this too is a sacred place.

Darkness and quiet, what more is needed?

Patience.

Or more accurately, the learning of an extreme slowness that comes close to immobility.

Without acceptance of this slowness, success is impossible; without it, we cannot truly communicate with an infant.

Relaxing, accepting the slow pace, letting it take command—all this requires training.

As much for the mother as for those of us who attend her ...

Without experiencing this extreme slowness in our own bodies, it is impossible to understand birth.

Impossible to receive the newborn baby properly.

His time is so slow as to approximate no movement at all.

Ours is an agitation bordering on frenzy.

Besides, "we are never truly here"—"always elsewhere."

In the past, with our memories; in the future, with our plans. Always before "or after." Never now.

But "we must learn to be here."

To forget the future, to forget the past.

Once again, everything is very simple.

And yet so hard to achieve.

How is it to be accomplished?

Only with the most passionate attention.[40]

Leboyer is saying that for those close to the birth, meditation becomes a natural response to the wombchild's energy, that it's worth devoting the most passionate meditative attention to the near-stillness of the child, an inconceivably dynamic near-stillness. The child so deeply needs to take its own time. We understand this when currently the child's timing is destroyed by induction in the large majority of U.S. births. Let Leboyer be a reminder that not being sensitive to the energy needs of the wombchild may be dangerous to childbirth health. By not recognizing the energy systems of the child, prevalent OB practice refuses to look for damage to the child's energy body systems.

In 1978 Leboyer published the book *Inner Beauty, Inner Light: Yoga for Pregnant Women.*[41] Today prenatal yoga courses are appreciated by pregnant women throughout the world, and Dr. Leboyer is somewhat responsible for that. Two of the traditional yoga *asanas* are sitting meditation and reclining meditation, *dhyana asana* and *savasana*. Those two yoga postures may have an even deeper impact on prenatal care. All of the traditional yoga *asanas* are based on a *pranic* body model, a body of energy power centers and meridians of energy flow.

Meditation Woman Speaks for Womankind

In 1974, the year of the publication of Leboyer's *Birth without Violence*, a twenty-five-year-old woman and mother of three published a book about the potential of natural childbirth and the importance of meditative discipline in prenatal care: *Prenatal Yoga and Natural Childbirth.* Jeannine Parvati Baker's language is superb. She became the first woman's voice of childbirth, and she shows us pregnancy as a path of human development, loaded with illumination potential. She learned Zen Buddhist meditation when she was a teenager, and later practiced both Buddhist and Hindu meditation methods. Jeannine developed a connection with energy breathing, which she used in her own births. Following are excerpts from her book:

Giving birth is initiation into women's mysteries ... It prepares us for other altered states and dying to the self. Giving conscious birth is a woman's vision quest, par excellence.... Opening for conscious birth helps all power centers to open.[42]

With breath as an ally we can receive a vision that will spiritually feed us our entire lives, right at the moment of conception and birth.[43]

... new and powerful feelings and levels of consciousness brought about by being pregnant ... Women talk of their childbirth experiences being transcendent, mystical, and/or the most profound spiritual experiences of their lives.[44]

Discipline is very much needed during pregnancy, not only from the ritual aspect, but to prepare for the great discipline required in caring for a baby.[45]

[Later, referring to yoga teacher Hari Dass] I thanked him for the advice to concentrate on my navel chakra during labor as this transformed labor pains into the gifts they really are.[46]

At the White Hole dimension of awareness, the personal dissolved and boundaries of self/other poured inside out with each birth-force wave. "Contractions" or labor pains were transformed into "gifts." Balancing between pleasure and pain brought power— power to be wisely used for the work at hand.[47]

Tremendous release when the baby emerges—like pulling the universe through the eye of a needle.[48]

Jeannine's three natural childbirths all spontaneously used energy breathing. Jeannine once said to me that she was channeling from the earth how to integrate childbirth and meditation. Her books and her work as a popular midwife and educator led the way to childbirth meditation and energy practice in childbirth.

Through meditation techniques that are now more widely available, more and more women find as Jeannine did that meditation helps them access instinctive wisdom and a new sense of body for birth.

31

The Use of Energy Meditation in Medicine

The use of mind-body methods in childbirth in the twentieth century can be said to have begun with the work of Dick-Read and Lamaze. Then mind-body medicine came of age. The use of energy medicine emerged. It advanced mind-body science.

For medicine in general, Dean Ornish made an important use of yogic breathing in his renowned heart care program. "In this system," he said, "we inhale not only oxygen but also energy, or *prana*. In Sanskrit, *prana* means both breath and spirit … breath is the vehicle for *prana* … These techniques … can expand the availability of energy to you."[49]

Dr. Ornish was using a model of the human body taken from Eastern medical and meditation traditions. He encouraged people to extend their sense of what they could do by breathing oxygen and energy at once, something they were made to do. The practice of energy breathing was revolutionary for people in his program. They were encouraged to relate to their body as a body of energy functions. That helped them see their bodies in a new way. They learned to practice energy medicine for themselves. The program and Dr. Ornish's book *Dr. Dean Ornish's Program for Reversing Heart Disease* were widely acclaimed.

Giving Birth in a Body Bright with Life

I've recently heard scientists speak with excitement about the dynamic function of the human body as if it had powerful internal radiation and luminosity. They said that the body has about ten billion cells that each have perhaps one hundred thousand chemical reactions per second. They said that a single human cell can emit up to ten thousand biophotons per second, communicating with the whole living system.* Photons are units of light.† The cellular photon emissions are essential

---

*Alexander Gurwitsch, "Z and Consciousness," YouTube, 2012, https://www.youtube.com/watch?v=ag6-JEGzzHc.
†Albert Einstein, "The Photoelectric Effect," 1905; Nobel Prize, 1921.

to our massive internal communications. At the same time, the vast systems of chemical reactions in the body emit bioluminescence, which is essential to other functions.

Evolving science lets us see more and more what the body is. The more we see, the more we're amazed at what we are. Subtle body physics is seeing increasing evidence of the radiant energy body structures described in ancient science.

It looks like today's woman has a marvelous body to give birth in.

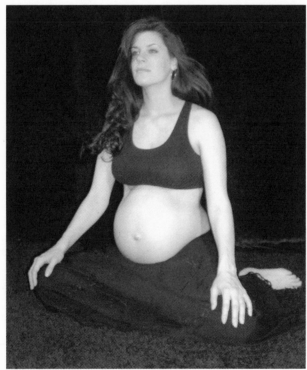

Photo by Patti Ramos

IV

Pregnancy as a Path of Human Development and Evolution

Now we've all heard of yogis of the East and practitioners of certain mystical disciplines who have been able, through breath training, to alter their perception of physical pain. Other people, known as mothers, demonstrate mastery equal to that of the yogis, when with proper training... they use breathing techniques to control pain in childbirth.

—Candace Pert[50]

The Liberation of the Womb

Carlos Castaneda introduced the term "energy body" in his remarkable series of books about the Toltec lineage of Mexico. His teacher, don Juan Matus, spoke of the traditional knowledge of the superiority of the woman's body, both in energy body and physical body design:

> According to don Juan Matus, one of the most specific interests of the shamans who lived in Mexico in ancient times was what they called the "liberation of the womb." He explained that the liberation of the womb entailed the awakening of its secondary functions, and that since the primary function of the womb, under normal circumstances, was reproduction, [they] were solely concerned with what they considered to be its secondary function: evolution. Evolution, in the case of the womb, was, for them, the awakening and full [use] of the womb's capacity to process direct knowledge... Females can see energy directly more readily than males because of the effect of their wombs... Women, because they have a womb, are so versatile, so individualistic in their ability to see energy directly

that this accomplishment, which should be a triumph of the human spirit, is taken for granted.[51]

There are several truths here giving further meaning to what has been called the natural superiority of women.[52] Most women have an inherent ability to see energy. This is an extraordinary advantage in meditation practices in which vital essences in the air are sensed and breathed into the energy body for greater function.

The second significant advantage for the woman in traditional meditation practices that focus on breathing into the lower abdomen is that the womb can "process direct knowledge." It's called the secondary womb function but clearly it's a great cognitive resource that might be used in the primary womb function, reproduction.

The Navel Center as a Natural Focus of Meditation

Dr. Cheng Man Ch'ing (1902–75) was the most distinguished grandmaster of Chinese medicine and T'ai Chi of the twentieth century. He moved to New York for the first time in 1963 and had a strong presence there intermittently until his death. He published important medical books, including texts on gynecology and obstetrics. He also taught T'ai Chi as a healing art. He was a remarkable doctor of the energy body–physical body dynamic.

In his book *Cheng Tzu's Thirteen Treatises on T'ai Chi Ch'uan* (1985), Ch'ing states that beginners who start to learn T'ai Chi Ch'uan should secure their mind and chi* in the tan tien. They must "sink the *chi* into the *tan tien*." In his book, *chi* is sometimes translated as "breath." The tan tien is located in the center of the energy body. The center of the tan tien is behind the umbilicus, closer to the navel than the spine.

When sinking the *chi* into the *tan tien*, the breathing must be fine, long, quiet and slow. Gradually inhale into the *tan tien* [breathe

* "*Qi* [*Chi*] is fundamental to Chinese medical thinking, yet no one English word or phrase can adequately capture its meaning. Perhaps we can think of *Qi* as matter on the verge of becoming energy or energy at the point of materializing" (Ted J. Kaptchuk, *The Web That Has No Weaver*, New York: Congdon and Weed, 1983, 35).

into the energy body]. The *chi* stays with the awareness. Then day after day, and month after month, the *chi* accumulates, naturally, without being forced. This accumulated *chi* is power for living more completely.[53]

This is a good practice for pregnancy. Focusing chi into the tan tien is focusing life-giving energy toward the womb. "Sinking the *chi* into the *tan tien* can give each internal organ its own exercise and stimulation for proper function."[54]

There are various traditional forms of T'ai Chi. Cheng Man Ch'ing's was an "internal energy" form. Both for organ health and greater function, T'ai Chi is excellent for prenatal care, offering an expanded vision of body and movement.

Judyth O. Weaver, PhD, who had studied Zen meditation in Japan, became a T'ai Chi Ch'uan student and patient of Cheng Man Ch'ing upon her return to New York in 1968 and has written eloquently about her use of T'ai Chi during pregnancy and birth:

When I became pregnant in 1970 I was overjoyed and felt that t'ai chi ch'uan would be my support during my pregnancy. Without question I intuitively knew it was the best exercise for me during this time and that it would help me stay limber and relaxed and in touch with the changes I would be going through. I was correct about all those intuitions.

It was fascinating tuning into myself every day as my body changed and as my belly became larger and my balance altered to answer the various developments. It was the daily meditation and moving that kept me attuned to all that was happening and all that I needed to respond to.

Spending as much time as I could at Shr Jung while I was pregnant was a very supportive experience. Classes were wonderful and I never had a problem with my growing, changing body. I was sure it was the best activity for me to do during this incredibly potent, important time and everyone there was helpful and supportive.

I am a very small person, have never been taller than 5 feet, and the baby I was carrying grew very large. People would stop me on the street and ask if I was carrying twins or triplets. The bulge in front of me grew unusually large. I was told I looked as if I had swallowed a very large watermelon. Yet I was also told that I was so graceful and carried myself (and my baby) elegantly. The t'ai chi was serving me well in so many ways.

I assumed that I was an earth mother and would birth in a very easy manner. Unfortunately all did not work out as I hoped. But t'ai chi helped me nonetheless. While I was in labor and had back pain t'ai chi supported me throughout the process. Every time I had to get up and relieve my bladder (and that was very often) I did the first section of the form and the pain was also relieved. The birthing process turned out to be an emergency caesarian section, partially, the doctor said, because my daughter was so big. After that shock it was time to do t'ai chi again. The medical professionals were surprised to find me standing and moving around and were amazed at my quick recovery and my ability to care for my infant even so immediately after major surgery.[55]

Judyth Weaver's story reveals the power of her deeper sense of body and function coming from sinking chi into her navel center during pregnancy and birth. The practice helped her heal from the side effects of medicines and surgery and helped her stay empowered through a very challenging birth.

Hara, the Vital Center

Zen meditation in Japan, transmitted from the Ch'an lineage of China, also features breathing into the navel center. The method is defined and explored in Karlfried Graf Von Dürckheim's book *Hara*. The *hara*, "the honored middle," known as the primal center, contains the tan tien, a focal point for meditation located two inches below the navel. Breathing into the tan tien is "right earthing," and opens the treasure of life. Von Dürckheim writes:

Sitting... [into] the *Hara*-seat not only refers to the position and weight of the belly within the whole body but also suggests the whole mood of stable sitting. This stability implies at once an outward and an inward balance: it means that the inner center is situated in the right place in the physical body, as well as the right placing of the center of gravity within the body... When the belly is sedate* the center is situated below.[56]... Breathing is once more easy and free, and a pleasant feeling arises from below.[57]... What is necessary is a movement which leads downwards to the all-dissolving, all absorbing depth of the Source.[58]

This is a naturally healthy and right practice for pregnancy. Breathing down into her vital navel center, the woman breathes into the depth of the Source.

How important can sitting meditation be for pregnant women today, living with continuing high levels of stress and uncertainty, at a fast pace?

With [breathing into the] *Hara* the uprightness of the body is no longer the result of will and power but comes by itself. The whole body finds itself in flexible equilibrium. The difference in the tension of the neck is a special criterion of right posture. It is as if a secret power soared up lightly from below and culminated in the free carriage of the head. And so the letting go above gives concentration of strength below and the resulting easy freedom of the head has its counterpart in the sustaining weight of the trunk. Thus the practice of [breathing into the] *Hara* consists from the beginning in a constantly repeated letting go or dropping down movement. Then one notices how from the vital middle region strength rises straight upward through the back and produces the sensation of being uplifted.[59]

Through the centuries, for pregnant women in both Chinese and Japanese meditation traditions, sitting meditation practice has offered remarkable birth enhancement. According to Von Dürckheim, "The exercise of sitting is the most fundamental of all. Here the practice of stillness has its source. A thousand secrets are known in simply sitting still."[60] We can see that sitting meditation can be a superior means of preparing for conscious childbirth.

---

* In *Webster's New World Dictionary and Thesaurus*, the word "sedate" translates into not excitable, composed, calm (1992, 342).

Feeding Elixir into the Child

Much ancient wisdom about the potential of deep breathing is contained in the Zen classic *The Embossed Tea Kettle* by the Zen Master Hakuin Zenji:

> As has been said by ancient wise men, the elixir is below the navel, the fluid is the fluid of the lungs, and one turns down the fluid of the lungs to the space below the navel, and so turns the lung fluid into the elixir.[61]

The "fluid" in the lungs is the vital energy breathed into the body from the air,[62] "turned down" (breathed down) into the vital area below the navel. The language in Hakuin's writing is the language of medicine, of restoring and perfecting health. His remedies were renowned for being effective. He continues:

> There are twelve kinds of breathings which help in curing all diseases. There is the rule about seeing a bean, as it were, below the navel. The purpose of doing so is to bring down the fire of the heart and concentrate it below the navel and right down to the soles of the feet. This not only cures diseases but helps greatly in Zen meditation.[63]

In this traditional wisdom about human capability, the fluid energy breathed down into the vital lower abdominal area is seen to be stored there and is naturally retained:

> There is what we call the "space below the abdomen" and this is the treasure room where the energy is stored and preserved; here is the fortress town where the divine elixir is purified so that life may be preserved for long years.[64]

When a pregnant woman practices breathing vital energy down to the child in her womb, she gives the child elixir for development, so that the child may have the potential of great and long life. The child will be blessed by such intention and could be interested in meditation. This can be seen as the basis of a healthy society.

Secret Instructions

In the book *The Secret of the Golden Flower,* a Chinese classic, translator Richard Wilhelm writes of the inner circulation of light and making breathing rhythmical. We might say that what he calls light is chi, a subtle protoplasm. He says that the circulation of the light is in unison with the rhythms of breathing. The breath, the heart, and the light are interdependent.

While in an upright sitting posture, an open channel is established that shifts the light downward, through the body, for circulation with the breath. This brings fine attention to the quality of breathing. There is more and more release in quieted consciousness.

True breathing, as Wilhelm refers to it, is manifested in the quietness of the breath, when you become more conscious of the work of the heart. Then the movement of the heart can be known. "As the breathing is light, the heart is light."[65]

The heart runs away easily, Wilhelm tells us, and it is necessary to bring it back to center through the power of breathing. When we refine the power of breathing, the heart becomes stable and quiet. Wilhelm addresses two mistakes of "quiet work": laziness and distraction. Sitting meditation posture will decrease distraction. Distraction often comes from letting the spirit wander aimlessly. Therefore, while sitting, it is helpful to keep the heart quiet with a concentrated attention and quiet breathing. The heart alone is conscious of the in- and out-flowing of the breath. The true breath cannot be heard with the ears.

When a pregnant woman practices breathing meditation to calm, she practices a greater form of body. She may feel she's preparing for a greater kind of birth.

The Life Vase and the Womb

Among the various methods of Vajrayana Buddhist meditation now well received in the West are practices that use the visualization of the Life Vase (*tse bum* in Tibetan), which is located in the human navel center, where the womb is in the physical body of a woman. It has also been called the Vase of Immortality.

The classic icons or buddha images of the Vajrayana each represent a different aspect of the human potential. One of the human buddha images is Amitayus, the Buddha of Infinite Life, sitting in meditation holding the Life Vase in his or her lap.

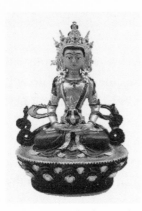

Amitayus is an androgynous buddha in human form whose radiant red energy body illuminates surrounding space. The buddha hands rest one in the other facing upright in the lap, holding the Vase of Life.

You can see by the way the image is formed that the Life Vase could also be inside the human buddha, centered in the

The Buddha of Infinite Life.   navel. The vase is rounded like the belly but it's in the energy body. The vase is an energetic form in the human body. It's in the same space as a womb in a woman. The illustration shows that the radiant red human Buddha of Infinite Life may be holding a wombchild in the Life Vase.

Based on my understanding of the physicists quoted in this book, the energy body and physical body are inseparable and unified in hyperspace. These bodies function at different frequencies of vibration. When the Buddha of Infinite Life is a pregnant woman, her womb slowly develops upward and moves into the same space as the energetic vase.

The meditation practice of vase breathing goes with this visualization. The pregnant woman doing the practice breathes life-giving chi into the Life Vase in her womb. She feeds the development of the child's powerful subtle body in her womb.

Pain-Body Release

A woman can bring a greater sense of her body and ability into labor and delivery if she recognizes her pain-body. She can release centuries of accumulated fear that may arise in her in childbirth. Eckhart Tolle writes about the woman and her pain-body in his book *The Power of Now:*

> Every woman has her share in what could be described as the collective female pain-body. This consists of accumulated pain suffered by women partly through male subjugation of the female, through slavery, exploitation, rape, childbirth, child loss, and so on, over thousands of years ... Often, a woman is "taken over" by the pain-body ...[66]

This challenge would tend to be there for most women during labor and delivery. The woman is apt to lose herself in the psychic pull of billions of women who have suffered in childbirth, and many thousands suffering at that moment, unless she has developed meditation awareness in preparation for labor. Then she may awaken to fully engage childbirth, avoiding the pull of suffering, able to stay free by appreciating contraction pain, realizing greater function:

> Do not let the pain-body use your mind and take over your thinking. Watch it. Feel its energy directly, inside your body. As you know, full attention means full acceptance.[67]

Women have the inherent ability to acknowledge the pain-body and not react to it, to not be disturbed by it, to appreciate the sensations of cervical opening. Whether they use this natural capability or not is an educational challenge for society since our system strongly approves of the use of powerful pharmaceutical drugs in childbirth instead of helping women access their inherent ability. Education in natural pain management and human development could inspire a new sense of body and ability in pregnant women.

When a woman in labor is aware of the collective pain-body and does not succumb to it, but sees it and frees it in the realization potential of labor, she can help free the species of its past and live its evolution. If she intends that, she can do that, and she can learn to intend that. Give women an educated chance. Pregnant women can practice safeguarding the great potential of the human species.

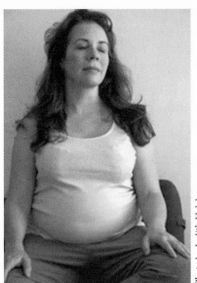

Photo by Judith Halek

V

The Calm Birth Method

I know now that human beings are creatures of awareness, involved in an evolutionary journey of awareness, beings indeed unknown to themselves, filled to the brim with incredible resources that are never used ...

—Carlos Castaneda[68]

Emerging Childbirth Methods

It is time to go deeper into the potential of childbirth methodology, starting with natural birth practice. We know enough about medical birth practice to know that it's expensive and risky, with potential long-term consequences affecting health, and its costs are high because of malpractice lawsuits.[69] We do not know enough about the potential of noninvasive childbirth methods.

In the twentieth century, we had several natural childbirth methods, all incorporating some use of mind-body practice. In the twenty-first century, our sense of the human body and potential has advanced. Mindfulness meditation, with its remarkable record in pain and anxiety management, and energy meditation are both being used by women wanting healthier childbirth. They hope that meditation will increase their chances of childbirth without medical interventions. Childbirth meditation certainly does that, given its capacity to enhance immune functioning, speed healing, and help to maintain present moment awareness in the face of challenges. It is also the healthiest way to have a medical birth. Emerging childbirth methodology has the potential to give us high standards of maternal and infant health.

Calm Birth is an example of emerging childbirth practice. Refined through twenty years of development and application, the Calm Birth method offers complete breathing and increased function in childbirth, making it possible for women to access their inherent potential for extraordinary experience in giving birth. Calm Birth offers a chance to regain a sense of the sacred in childbirth, whether or not medical interventions are used. Intention is integral to Calm Birth, the intention to benefit life by giving birth in a greater way.

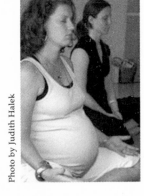

Photo by Judith Halek

There are three practices in the method:

» Practice of Opening
» Womb Breathing
» Giving and Receiving

These practices are described in detail in the following pages.

Calm Birth Practice One: Practice of Opening

Calm Birth is based on the clinical and research programs in the medical uses of meditation of the Harvard Medical School (HMS) and the University of Massachusetts Medical Center (UMMC). In the UMMC medical meditation program, designed to treat difficult medical cases in which pain management is often a primary concern, a combination of three practices has proved effective since 1979: reclining meditation, sitting meditation, and awareness-movement exercises. The Calm Birth program is similar to the UMMC program in that it uses three practices: reclining meditation, sitting meditation, and a renowned healing practice.

Regarding the reclining meditation, UMMC uses the celebrated method of progressive relaxation (PR) developed by Edmund Jacobson, MD, at the Harvard Medical School and the University of Chicago Medical School, from the 1920s into the 1940s. The method often causes neuromuscular release and nervous system healing, successfully treating various disease conditions. UMMC combines PR with mindfulness meditation, which makes the neuromuscular release more efficient. Calm Birth uses neuromuscular release with mindfulness and modifies it for childbirth for the following purposes:

» To practice the healing of the nervous systems of woman and wombchild in preparation for childbirth. The nervous system of the fetus may be healed of prenatal disturbances and adverse neural conditions by sympathetic resonance with the woman's progressive neuromuscular release.

» To engage life force at the cellular level, to increase vitality in preparation for childbirth.

» To directly engage the wombchild for prenatal development.

PR methods are an early and valuable form of mind-body medicine. PR has provided impressive evidence of its effectiveness in successfully treating: acute neuromuscular hypertension, chronic neuromuscular hypertension, states of fatigue and exhaustion, states of debility (convalescence from infectious and exhausting diseases of various types), organic and functional coronary disorders, chronic pulmonary tuberculosis, preoperative and postoperative conditions, toxic goiter, insomnia, various internal spasm conditions, including cardiospasm, and other conditions. This is proven mind-body medicine.

Dr. Jacobson saw that neuromuscular release therapy depended on patient self-initiative and nervous system reeducation. This was a breakthrough in noninvasive medicine and self-care, verging into new kinds of treatment. Jacobson developed extensive variations of PR in his medical practice.

The UMMC program uses a forty-five-minute reclining body scan to achieve progressive relaxation. Hundreds of American hospitals now use the UMMC reclining method with proven success. By combining mindfulness meditation with PR, the mind is often successfully prevented from wandering, so that attention is kept valuably focused from moment to moment, maximizing effectiveness of the practice. The body scan brings neuromuscular release and restoration.

With respect to prenatal care, mindfulness-based PR offers a superior kind of relaxation meditation that may rectify existing conditions and enable women to reach deep resource.

The Calm Birth program applies mindfulness-based progressive relaxation for childbirth with an emphasis on developmental communion with the wombchild and contact with life force at the cellular level. The Practice of Opening leads women through a process of neural reconditioning that prepares them for optimal function during delivery, for the giving of life.

The Practice of Opening may bring extraordinary pre-birth experience and near-birth experience, make paranormal experiences more accessible because awareness is less restricted by nervous stresses, and is supported by hormonal enhancements, as described in Chapter II of this book.

Key Points

» Practice of Opening offers rest, restoration, and release for increased natural capability during labor and delivery.

» The relaxing of neuromuscular tensions and rectifying conditions caused by stress deepens confidence and awareness.

» By doing Practice of Opening, a woman may experience relief from long-standing health challenges while she takes superior prenatal care.

» This method can bring the pregnant woman and her partner into healing and a healthful union with the child, an awareness cohesion that should enhance the child's intelligence.

» The experience of inner light may be one of our earliest and most fundamental experiences. In Practice of Opening, women directly engage light in their body as prenatal resource.

» Practice of Opening is intended to give women a healing method for self-empowerment and personal development in preparing to give birth.

» Childbirth has often been a time of extraordinary experience for women, including spiritual and paranormal experience. Practice of Opening encourages such events.

» Practice of Opening is a reclining PR meditation intended to bring the awareness of the woman into communion with the awareness of the wombchild, and to help women discover new kinds of ability in preparing to give birth.

» The practice is performed by listening to the Calm Birth audioguide (CD or MP3), available via www.calmbirth.org.

The Method

Choose a quiet place dedicated to childbirth meditation. It can be the bedroom if necessary. If so, use blankets or mats on the floor.

Use the bed as a last resort. It's important to not fall asleep in the reclining practice. Use blankets and pillows as needed to be comfortable. You need to be at rest and alert with soft open eyes.

The audioguide helps the woman be present in her body feeling the great action of her living systems. Beginning with sensing her life force directly, her attention is focused to move progressively through her body, to release neuromuscular stresses and recondition her nervous system. The muscle systems are progressively relaxed, taking pressure off the nervous system and the organs, allowing inner alignment and cognitive enhancement in the woman and child. When a partner or other supporter joins in this practice, bonding with the child in the womb, the child's vital energy and awareness potentially increase. Partner benefits include: being part of the birth experience and being more prepared for birth.

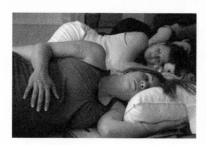 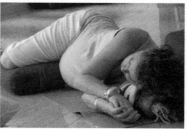

Photo by Judith Halek

The Practice (the audioguide, line by line)

Practice of Opening is a reclining meditation.

It offers a way to progressively relax and open your body,

releasing stress on your nerves,

to practice healing your nervous system.

The wombchild is responsive to meditation

in both mother and father.

This practice is a chance to come into greater awareness,

to enliven you and your child.

You're a woman holding new life dynamically alive in your womb,

or you're a man who wants to benefit your partner and child

by imagining the womb in yourself.

With this practice you learn to rest and release,

gaining vital strength and new function.

Please find a comfortable place to rest

and lie down mindfully, using pillows as needed.

It's important to be comfortable and warm.

This practice is done with soft open eyes

so that you don't fall asleep.

The effects are immediate, and they build over time.

You'll benefit the most with daily practice.

Whenever you need to rest, this is an ideal way

to calm and open your body

and enter the life force in your cells.

[The Practice]

Please take a deep breath, deep into life, and exhale slowly.

Feel life energy in all of your body at once.

Again breathe deep into life, and exhale easily.

Let yourself experience total body sensation.

Feel the action of billions of cells and energy flows.

Please imagine the dynamics of your central nervous system,

taking care of countless functions at once.

Messages travel quickly to and from your developing child.

Rest, and understand that as you become

aware of living light in you,

you directly benefit the child in your womb.

From head to toes feel your body's flow.

Experience the enlivening of your child.

Feel that the new life in you is unlimited.

Feel the living presence of your child.

As your awareness expands

take time to relax, slowly and deeply, resting in union.

Soon you'll be guided to focus part by part into your body,

to release all that needs to be released.

As you breathe, open and sense all the life moving

in you and your child.

Every time you return to this awareness

you feel great internal life support.

Feel the forces creating life in you, sustaining life in you.

Recognize the miracle of life you are,

and the miracle of life being created in you,

the child in your womb.

Now notice the toes of both your feet.

Experience the life in your toes.

Feel their energy channels.

Feel the energy channels in your feet.

Throughout your feet notice how the bones give stability and form.

Sense how your feet serve you in many ways.

If there's any discomfort, notice where.

Breathe into it and release as much as you can.

Feel the total current of life in your feet.

Move your attention up into the calves of both your legs.

Sense the intertwined muscles, blood vessels, and nerves.

Sense how the muscles, nerves, and blood flow all work together.

Sense how muscle tension impacts your flows.

Throughout your feet and lower legs,

feel and relax more muscle stress on your nerves.

Feel an increase of vitality in your lower legs and feet.

Now become aware of your knees.

Notice life force moving through them.

This is a good way to meditate, reclaiming your body,

knowing your body as if for the first time, a body alive with child.

From your knees, come up into your thighs.

Feel how your living thighs support and carry your body.

Notice and release any tension in your buttocks.

Recognize their power to support you in childbirth.

All throughout your feet, legs, and hips,

feel the smaller and larger bones,

muscles, blood vessels, and nerves.

Feel it all together.

Release any holding.

Feel the energy gain and sense the life flow.

As you feel your body and your child more and more

you both become more alive.

It is time to bond directly.

Place your hands lightly on your belly.

Be sensitive to the life of your child.

Feel the life force in you both.

Come into new life in your self and your child.

Release any block to the full flow of life.

Enter greater awareness.

Sense the power and wisdom of your child.

If you feel tension, breathe into it, and give it space.

Breathe into and out of any areas of discomfort or pain.

Please relax more and more.

Feel both of your arms full of life.

Feel life force moving through your arms and hands.

Rest your wrists and relax your hands.

Feel their healing ability.

Imagine their potential to care for your child.

Relaxing your arms down through your fingers,

breathe care into the child,

trusting the process of life.

Feel your womb and cervix holding your child.

At the right time, your womb will start to flex

and your cervix will begin to respond,

slowly opening, progressively releasing new life.

The baby's head will then move down through the birth canal.

The pelvis will work with the womb

when you breathe the baby down to be born.

Feel the strength and flexibility of your womb,

yielding to growth and change.

These are the strongest muscles in your body,

fully capable of birthing your baby.

Relax any abdominal tension caused by anxiety.

Feel the perfect hold of the muscles that cradle your child.

Surrender into the full support of life.

Trust your ability to change.

Prepare to GIVE birth to your child.

Now, turning your focus to your baby, envision your child's head,

facial features, torso, arms and legs, muscles, nerves.

See your child's heart pulsing blood and light all through its body,

feeding the cells with radiant life.

It's time to feel the nurturing flow of your organs

and the energetic organs of your child.

Feel the flow of life in your flesh,

and practice sensitivity to the energies of the child.

Trust the living wisdom in you both.

Now please turn your attention to the umbilical cord and placenta,

vibrant with thousands of body processes.

Imagine the energy flowing in the lifelines of the cord,

back and forth between your child's body

and your nurturing placenta.

All around this is the cradling womb.

Once again feel your whole body,

deeper and more completely than ever.

Breathe awareness into your belly.

Breathe easily and deep,

bringing in oxygen and energy.

As you breathe out, gently contract your belly inward,

caressing your child.

Recognize any abdominal tension from anxiety restricting your breath.

Let the muscles there release. Trust the flow of life.

Completely open yourself to your body.

Completely open yourself to your baby.

Completely open yourself to life.

Breathe easily and deep.

Please bring your attention into your upper body.

Relax the muscles through your rib cage and chest.

Notice any fear.

Please recognize and release any stress.

Trust your ability and strength.

Open your shoulders and chest.

Breathe in deeply, and relax as you exhale.

Feel your breasts coming alive with milk.

Know that your breasts are vital for your child.

As you continue breathing for you both,

enter the dynamic majesty of your heart.

Recognize all that the heart does to maintain life.

Intuit your heart's fourfold pulsing rhythm.

It beats for every cell in you and your child.

Your heart sustains your lives.

Open into pulsing union.

Rest in pulsing union.

Bring your focus to your back.

Let your spine extend.

Feel bones and connective tissue adjust.

The life force in your spine

carries you and your child.

Please bring your awareness up your spine,

through your shoulders into your neck.

Open and let sensation flow.

The stress of demands of the day

often tighten the neck and head.

Let your neck and head relax together.

Let yourself be free right now.

Feel your breath flowing in, and flowing out.

Now, become aware of your face.

Breathe into your jaw letting it loosen.

Notice the different sets of muscles around your mouth,

for all your conscious and unconscious expressions.

Find all these muscles and relax them,

releasing all expression.

Let your mouth open a little

and release any holding in your lower face and neck.

Relax your tongue and silently flow.

Come to your eyes and the muscles that surround them.

Sense all the expression they could have,

all the expression of your life.

Relax all that completely. Let it go.

Prepare to feel empowered giving birth.

Let your face be free right now.

Resting with soft open eyes,

your energized body prepares.

This is an empowerment path.

To conclude the practice,

know that you've blessed yourself and your child.

Live in this awareness as you move.

Calm Birth Practice Two: Womb Breathing

Womb Breathing the Night of the Birth

Womb Breathing is energy breathing for childbirth. Energy breathing has been known and used for centuries. It's a natural ability, a kind of breathing most people are able to do when they're shown how. Energy breathing is complete breathing, breathing oxygen and vital energy.

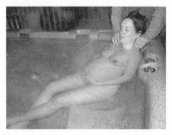

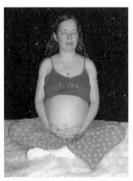

Debbie in tub, 9 cm dilation
(an hour before the birth).

Debbie at 5 cm dilation.

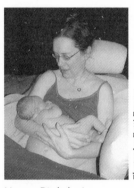

Happy Birthday!

Photos by Patti Ramos

During the history of our planet, in various cultures, meditation traditions developed in which breathing vital energy from the air into the navel center in the human energy system was a key feature. That was known to have great value for human development and evolution. Though the direction to breathe energy into the navel center was given regardless of gender, practitioners were predominantly men. Women were generally not expected to be interested in such practice, and were probably not encouraged to breathe vital energy. But in some situations, such as in the Nyingma lineage of Tibetan Buddhism, women and men were equally encouraged to breathe vital energy. And when the women practitioners were pregnant and did vase breathing, they knew they were giving the wombchild extraordinary prenatal care.

Womb Breathing is closely based on the Vajrayana Buddhist (Tibetan) meditation method called vase breathing (*bum chung* in Tibetan). *Bum chung* is "small vase breathing," or "gentle vase breathing," and is effortless. It is not to be confused with *bum chen*, "big vase breathing," which is intense, and not appropriate for childbirth preparation.

Because of the presence of Tibetan meditation masters in Europe and America during the past fifty years, the practice of bum chung has been available for use in childbirth in the West from an authoritative living tradition.

Energy breathing quiets the body and can bring calm into labor and delivery. It can help women be undisturbed by thoughts and emotions during labor. The practice helps women be open and receptive during contractions, and deeply calm in the intervals between contractions. Some of the women go through labor always aware of the child and the vase.

Partners in the birth, as well as midwives, nurses, doctors, and doulas, can practice breathing energy to be supportive of the woman's practice, especially because in many Calm Births the audioguide of the practice instruction is playing in the room. When a partner is supportively doing Womb Breathing meditation, the unified prenatal team can take their childbirth into a great start of life.

A woman can learn to practice Womb Breathing while she sleeps, to benefit the wombchild. This instruction is given in the Calm Birth teacher training program.

The woman who develops meditation skills for childbirth may be learning meditation for the rest of her life. Childbirth can open the path of meditation. After childbirth, Womb Breathing becomes vase breathing, for postnatal care and healing, and for an ongoing practice of empowered breathing.

Key Points

» Womb Breathing offers pregnant women a way to shift into greater function, to breathe completely.

» Womb Breathing allows pregnant women to breathe both vital energy and oxygen.

» Women are able to use the vital energy they breathe for child development.

» Complete breathing helps women keep calm no matter what happens in the mind.

» Womb Breathing is a direct practice of undisturbed birth.

» The women who practice Womb Breathing are able to use inherent ability with developmental impact in the womb.

» Womb Breathing can be learned as three steps to power in pregnancy.

The Method

Womb Breathing is a sitting meditation practice based on a profound energy breathing technique proven effective for centuries. The practice works through respect for the innate ability of the human body and its extraordinary breathing potential. The practice of Womb Breathing can improve the quality of breathing and the quality of psychophysical activity, with important benefits for the child.

Psychologically, the practice is based on recognizing the difference between mind and awareness. This is mindfulness meditation, in which women learn to recognize their mind. While the women breathe energy, they train themselves to be aware of their mind, to see how laden with anxiety and fear it often is. They learn to recognize anxiety and fear and not react. They learn to see it and free it. They learn to calm their mind down. Women who practice this method become progressively more able to recognize and release anxiety and fear in childbirth, without being disturbed by it. These women practice psychologically undisturbed birth, sane birth.

Daily prenatal practice of this sitting meditation enables a deeper kind of breathing that takes place effortlessly beyond the practice period, throughout the course of the day and night, because the body likes to function at the more optimal levels it was designed for. Though this is a sitting practice, it naturally integrates into the natural movements of labor and birth.

Womb Breathing is the most essential of the three Calm Birth prenatal practices because it is complete breathing that may arise spontaneously at any time, coming from within, and may be of great value to women throughout the labor process. This sitting practice is based on visualization.

Visualization

Visualization can be transformative. Visualization of our body systems, such as our energy systems, can help people see the way to extraordinary activity.

If we visualize a pregnant woman's body as inseparable physical and energy systems, envisioning her breathing organs we can see her lungs in her chest and a luminous Life Vase in her navel energy center. The Life Vase is very near her womb, but in a different dimension. Physical science today might say that the Life Vase and the womb are in the same space in hyperspace in the body. The Life Vase is an important feature of the energy system in both women and men. It's made for a profound kind of breathing, to strengthen life force.

When a pregnant woman is practicing Womb Breathing, it may look like she's breathing into her womb, but actually she's breathing into her Life Vase to benefit the wombchild. She's using her full breathing capability, breathing with her physical and energy systems at once. With Womb Breathing, the woman uses her lungs fully, with abdominal breathing for full oxygenation, and she's simultaneously using her energy channel system by breathing energy into her vase. The energy breathed feeds up into her central psychic channel, for the optimal activity of the woman and the child in her womb.

As a woman spends more time engaged in the Womb Breathing practice, she can visualize and see her energy centers and channels more completely. Tradition tells us that the human energy system consists of countless channels, ranging in size from the large central psychic channel, with its radiant series of power centers, to small, fine conduits. The woman can see that her central energy channel rises from the bottom of the vase in her navel. She can see that she's made to breathe life-giving energy into the vase, which both stores energy and sends it up the central channel, to balance the energy centers and bring higher systems to life. This increased inner activity benefits the child in the womb through the child's neurohormones and through sympathetic resonance, the child's energetic response to the woman's energy uptake. First the woman imagines this, visualizing it as she practices it, but then most women are able to see their energy bodies more and more.

The whole system of channels is dynamic, and has been sensed, seen, and used by meditation science in different cultures for more than two thousand years. There are major and finer energy channels, and subtle channels that quickly pulse into and out of existence, depending on the energy states of the individual. The central energy channel with its brilliant power centers has energetic correspondence to the central nervous system, as the Life Vase corresponds to the womb in women.

The vase is located behind the physical navel, between four finger widths above the navel to four finger widths below. The central channel rises from the bottom of the vase up to the crown chakra power center located in the top of the head. The conscious breathing of the energy and physical bodies into dynamic cohesion is based on practical knowledge refined over many centuries.

Womb Breathing is vase breathing practiced by a pregnant woman. She knows that the Life Vase and the womb are interconnected. She visualizes and feels that the deep breathing practice benefits the womb-child energetically, biologically, and psychologically.

To visualize what is breathed, the woman senses that the air she lives in is in a universal energy field (UEF). The UEF is presently an important subject of scientific inquiry, but it has been recognized and utilized for more than two thousand years by important meditation science traditions. The UEF has been called universal chi and universal prana. Some scientists today call it protoplasm, the basis of living matter. The UEF is known to be omnipresent vital energy, and we're made to breathe it down into the vase. It has a fundamental affinity for the life in our bodies: inside the energy body, flowing in its channels, is the same fundamental vital energy. It's been called internal chi, internal prana. Most people can learn to sense it. The traditional medical sciences of acupuncture and acupressure work with it.

The external chi can be seen by some people but is mostly sensed. Women may sense it more quickly than men. Most people live their lives breathing it in and breathing it out without sensing or using it, without accessing its energetic potential.

Visualize the life-giving substance in the air and sense it. See it and breathe it and intend it down into the vase. You can feel yourself inhale it, intend it, and breathe it down into the vase directly, and you feel it go right through into the vase. You breathe the fine, life-giving substance in, intend it in and down, and you feel it go into the vase. From the vase it absorbs up into the central channel for more optimal mind-body action.

Knowledge that is considered sacred states that the energy body forms simultaneously with the physical body from conception. When it comes to visualizing her energy body, a woman may start to see with inner vision. She may visualize herself birthing for the greater good.

Posture

To experience the full benefit of Womb Breathing, it's important to sit so that the body is upright, comfortable, and balanced, on a cushion or in a chair. Sit with respect for the life force in you. If you can sit on the floor, it's good to sit cross-legged, using a cushion to lift the pelvis and sacrum, and bring the knees down, so the body weight is distributed evenly. The spine should be as upright as possible, balanced and at ease; it may tend to lift a little, effortlessly. When sitting in a chair, sit forward a little with your spine balanced as upright as possible. Both feet rest flat on the floor directly in front of you. Hands are placed on the knees, or cupped one in the other in the lap.

Sitting upright and balanced is the best posture for Womb Breathing. The woman can shift into spontaneous Womb Breathing in any posture, but sitting is the best posture for sustained, effective practice. It encourages coming to still-point to shift to awareness of the energy body. Sitting to come into greater operation enables women to calm down their minds and bring awareness down to the vital center.

Complete Breathing

Today's physical science, with its mighty instruments and spacecraft, looks into unlimited space and what do we see? We see that space is full of life-giving universal energy, an energy bank from which the universe evolves. This life-giving energy may be in several states at once, pervading all space. It is omnipresent energy-matter that perennial wisdom says is vital for life, and it's made to be breathed. All our life we've breathed that energy in and out without awareness and thus with inadequate absorption. The absorption is potentially under our control.

Awareness can direct the breathing of prana into the body. The external prana, vital life-energy of the universe, has an affinity for the life-giving prana in our fundamental nature. If that isn't recognized, then the energy is poorly absorbed. In Womb Breathing, that universal vital energy is recognized, breathed in, and intended directly into the Life Vase, for our energy system. It's done with an effortless deep breathing that also takes in maximum oxygen. And so this is complete breathing.

This fine, deep, slow breathing is rich in oxygen and energy. It's fine breathing because it senses and extracts fine substance from the air. It's deep breathing because it uses full breathing capability and brings the breath in deep, into the energy system. It's slow breathing because the increased intake requires fewer breaths per minute, expending less energy, increasing vital reserves, all so good for the woman and her wombchild.

Whatever posture the woman is in, it is important for her to breathe completely, using her belly, her chest, and her life vase breathing in a greater way. This kind of breathing can inspire women to breathe through any challenges that arise, to breathe free of any agony of mind that may arise. This kind of breathing helps pregnant women breathe free.

Controlled Release

In the traditional teaching of vase breathing, people are asked to practice a gentle retaining of the energy breathed down into the vase. Traditionally, people practice breathing energy down into the vase and then hold it briefly, for two or three seconds. They release the exhale before the retention feels uncomfortable.

Calm Birth has changed vase breathing a little with respect to pregnant women. To make vase breathing as easy as possible for pregnant women, we ask them to practice a controlled release, breathing energy effortlessly down into the vase, at ease in the normal cycle of breath, and then to exhale a little more slowly than inhaling.

Exhaling the vase breath a little more slowly than it is inhaled is practicing a gentle retaining of the vital energy. If there is the slightest discomfort or strain, the exhale can be immediately released. The woman can retain the breath as much as she wants to by spontaneously regulating how slowly or more quickly she wants to exhale.

It is generally effortless to exhale a little more slowly than one inhales, without disturbing the natural cycle of the breath. When the body is doing vase breathing on its own, naturally, it may gently retain the energy breath by exhaling slower than it inhales, giving the energy breathed into the vase a little more time to be absorbed up into the central energy channel.

Energy Increase from Breathing Energy

Womb Breathing sitting meditation saves, restores, and absorbs vital energy, giving birthing women inner strength and calm for fetal development, labor, and delivery. Sitting meditation slows the spending of energy in the ceaseless activity of life, giving women a method to stop the external action and calm down. In sitting meditation, energy reserves that may be run down from high activity levels begin to restore. Research has proved that meditation is significantly better than sleep for restoring and increasing energy.[70]

With Womb Breathing, women learn to shift frequently from mind to open awareness, saving vital energy that would be lost in the chaotic activity of mind. Mind burns up psychic energy. The willful feeding of energy to the mind is a primary cause of fatigue and burnout. Womb Breathing sitting meditation helps a woman free herself from the anxious action of the mind by repeatedly returning to open awareness, saving energy needed for greater function. Using a sitting meditation method to reduce the force of mind, women can have the energy and wisdom for the birth they want.

The shallow breathing prevalent in our anxiety-ridden era is inefficient, resulting in oxygen reduction and fatigue. It takes up to seven times more energy to breathe badly, overusing intercostal (between the ribs) muscles. Womb Breathing is effortless deep breathing, bringing in oxygen and energy with minimal energy cost.

With this more complete use of the human ability to breathe, a pregnant woman has the potential to give herself and her child the energy needed for vital health and full capability. For those who want to intentionally breathe life-giving energy, for those who want to breathe vital energy into their wombchild, universal vital energy has always been present for us to use.

Breathing into Contractions

Sometimes women stop breathing and hold their breath during contractions, or are directed to do shallow, high-chest, "pant-blow" breathing, which is like hyperventilation. That technique is admittedly useful at one critical juncture during labor, when it is desirable to stop an impulse to push at the point of crowning, in order to allow the perineal tissues to stretch to prevent tearing. Other than this case, both holding the breath and hyperventilation may cause fear by correspondence, because anxiety and fear most often cause people to hold their breath or to limit it to shallow, rapid breathing. Shallow breathing impedes oxygenation for woman and child. This inhibits both physiological and psychological capability in labor.

Breathing fully into contractions, something women are capable of but are too seldom encouraged to do, tends to reduce or eliminate the occurrence of fear, and gives women a positive, willed action to perform while the body continues the process of labor. Fear of pain intensifies the sensations and causes the body to work against itself through neuromuscular tension, thereby prolonging labor and often being the cause of medical intervention. Breathing into contractions reduces the incidence of fear and, therefore, medical intervention so that women can access their full range of ability in labor.

After practicing the shift from mind to awareness with Womb Breathing throughout pregnancy, women in labor tend to spontaneously deep-breathe into contractions. As a woman recognizes fear and frees herself to breathe, freeing her body to do its work, contraction pain is transformed as she breathes into it.

Following is a description by Gay Hendricks, PhD, of a birth he attended that demonstrated the innate capacity of a woman to breathe into contractions:

> …The laboring woman used her breath to breathe into the contractions, participating with the sensations rather than fighting them. By doing so she was able to transform the pain. Later she said it was never painful while she was using her breath. Sometimes a contraction would start as pain, but as she remembered to breathe into it, a shift would occur: Pain would become sensation.[71]

Clearly it's possible to breathe into contractions and remain undistracted in the process. A daily practice of energy breathing meditation supports this response.

Recognition and Release in Contractions

The key to staying undisturbed during contractions is adequate preparation in self-calming practices, such as Womb Breathing, on a daily basis, until the woman is prepared to see and let go of fear as it comes up. The more one practices psychological meditation such as Womb Breathing, the more one exposes mind to awareness. There are many aspects to the mind, one's own ordinary thinking, memories, and projections; but with respect to human development, anxiety and fear in the mind are what we need to wake up from. Particularly with respect to childbirth, when anxiety and fear can result in risky medical interventions that may impair fetal and/or maternal health, it is vital for women to know that they have methods available through which they can stop reacting to anxiety and fear. With Womb Breathing, women anticipate releasing fear in contractions. They're ready to recognize and release fear if it comes up.

Centuries of experience with meditation practices have shown that we have the innate capacity to recognize and release fear in its various forms, including anxiety. The more we practice meditation, the more we know the varieties of human anxiety and fear. Facing fear is transformative.

> The willingness to face fear is itself fearlessness. Fearlessness is not merely the numb absence of fear. It is the strength and dignity that are nourished each time we face fear directly... the strength that comes from directly stepping into fear... Each time you go directly through the gateway of fear, you touch a more profound level of fearlessness and genuine confidence.[72]

Facing fear changes its quality. That doesn't necessarily dispel it. But daily practice of mindful breathing meditation, such as Womb Breathing, makes it inevitable that pregnant women anticipate and catch their fears. They see that many and maybe all of the fears in them are not their own, but come from the collective unconscious mind. Fears that are more personally the woman's own are recognized as such and are energetically changed in that moment. Sometimes that's enough to dispel them.

The more we're aware of our mind, aware of our thoughts, the more we know we don't need to react to our thoughts. The more we're aware of our anxieties, the more we may stop feeding them. Meditation reduces the incidence of being disturbed by emotions. The woman who practices meditation for prenatal care is able to see and release anxieties that may arise in labor, to free herself and feel the species begin to heal.

Learning Complete Breathing

Learning to sense and breathe energy in the air and intend it down into the Life Vase can be compared to learning to ride a bicycle when you were a child. At first it may seem difficult—balancing on the bike, using the pedals, and moving ahead all at once—but seeing that all the other children learned how to do it was encouraging. Countless thousands of people have done energy breathing, for centuries, and now more and more people are doing it around you as the interest in meditation grows. Sensing that you were made to breathe completely, when you first breathe energy and intend it down into the vase and feel it go into the vase, you know something alive has happened and you're beginning to get the knack. Please apply patience and perseverance.

Establishing an Effective Practice

The effectiveness of Womb Breathing depends on the quality of the practice. Though critical mass is important—that is, the more the method is used, the better—there are two important factors: the quality of attention and the energy of intention. They are related, but not the same.

In general, the stronger the intention to raise the quality of one's meditation, the better one's attention tends to be, and the more effective the practice. A woman may have good-quality attention to the method for her first birth, and then find that through developments in her being, when she applies Womb Breathing for the second birth her intention is even stronger and the quality of her attention is even better. That tends to be the case. Or it can be that intention is strong, but individual life demands make attention difficult. In all cases patience and perseverance are needed.

The wider the scope of the intention of the practice, the better. The best energy of intention is to want to fully benefit yourself, your child, your family, your society, and your planet by raising the quality of your childbirth.

For Womb Breathing to be effective in labor, a daily practice is recommended. Women who establish a daily sitting practice develop biological well-being and psychological strength. They intentionally give the child the benefits of prenatal meditation and raise their level of awareness for making the right decisions during labor.

As important as diet is in pregnancy, there may be nothing more important women can do to take charge of their health and their birthing process than to practice meditation every day, to personally reduce stress. Women who meditate for childbirth generally have good diet discipline too. Daily morning practice is the best way to start the day, to enrich pregnancy and for personal development.

Practice as early in the morning as possible, to start the day in an empowering way. Find the quietest place available. Establish that as your regular place of practice. Your meditation energy will collect there and support you. If necessary, the place where you practice can be your bedroom.

As we have learned from advances of quantum physics, whatever we do does not just happen locally; it also occurs universally, simultaneously. What we do to improve the quality of life on our planet affects all life, inseparably, everywhere in the universe. For optimal practice of new childbirth methods based on self-care, such as Calm Birth, it's best to raise awareness and intention without limit.

A Daily Bedtime Commitment

The Calm Birth teacher training shows childbirth professionals how to do Womb Breathing before going to sleep in order to maintain the practice while asleep. The body likes to do Womb Breathing on its own. By holding the intention before falling asleep, people can naturally perform the practice without conscious involvement. Remarkable benefits may come. Sustained practice is often empowering, and can be transformative.

Instinctive Movement and Vocalization in Labor

The Calm Birth method, practiced with the intention to function at a higher level during childbirth, gives women a basis for confidence. One purpose of Calm Birth is to enable women to slow down and reach their inner core of being, where the birth energy flows, helping them ride it instinctively.

In accord with the published findings of Michel Odent, MD, and the perennial wisdom of midwives, the Calm Birth program affirms a woman's need for privacy, low light, spontaneous movement, and freedom to vocalize, to be undisturbed in labor.

> …Given the right kind of environment, where she could feel free and uninhibited … a woman could naturally reach a level of response [and resource] deeper within her than individuality, upbringing, or culture.[73]

There is no doubt that free movement in labor is an important need. Different kinds of maternal positions, suggested by the sensations of contraction and cervical opening, enable the baby to more easily find her or his way from the womb into the world. This lets the woman access a primal neural resource that knows how to lead her quickly and safely to birth. Laboring, pushing (if necessary), and giving birth from a standing or supported squatting position ("vertical birth") has been a choice of women for thousands of years. Waterbirth can be ideal for women. Warm water supports the woman's body and relaxes her, allowing her to birth vertically with minimum muscular tension. The child has lived only in liquid, so waterbirth offers a natural and gentle transition. The child arises from the water breathing oxygen from its mother through the umbilical cord.

Just as a birthing woman may need to move, or squat, or dance, she may need to use her voice. She may need to make sounds she's never made. She may need to make energy tones, some of them deep, resonant sounds. She may sing personal power, primal moan, and / or make sharper expressive calls, sometimes with rhythm. This is undisturbed birth, encouraging the woman to feel free. A woman who breathes energy for birth may at some point sing or shout energy through the contraction, undisturbed. No matter how intense it gets, the peace of complete breathing keeps coming back. Then, all the more, the force is with her.

Womb Breathing in Three Steps to Power

Step One: The Power of Sitting

Sit down into your body as if you're sitting into life itself.

Feel your balance and stability and lift.

Sit still to stop the world.

Sit into all your inner resource.

"A thousand secrets are revealed in sitting still."

Sit to come into your power.

Step Two: The Power of Awareness

Turn your attention to your breath.

Feel your body breathing itself.

Pay attention as you slowly breathe in,

and then breathe out, effortlessly, completing the cycle of breath.

Notice that at the end of the out-breath there's a gap,

a break, stillness to help you calm your mind.

Then your mind comes in powerfully and takes your attention away.

To regain awareness keep coming back to your breath.

You keep bringing attention back to awareness, free of mind.

Mind takes your attention away and awareness brings you back.

You can shift the power in you from mind to awareness.

You can bring yourself to life with awareness of breath.

Step Three: The Power of Complete Breathing

Step Three calms the mind even more deeply with *complete breathing*.

Women learn to breathe both oxygen and vital energy.

They learn to empower themselves with greater function in breathing.

Women learn to breathe life-giving energy that's always been in the air.

Using innate breathing ability, inborn resource,

the woman empowers herself with a more complete kind of care,

breathing life-giving energy into herself and her child.

The woman sees that the world has always been life-giving.

When mind and its fears arise, she tends to calm.

Such women access the power to have a greater kind of birth.

The Practice (the audioguide, line by line)

Womb Breathing is energy breathing for childbirth.

It gives you deep body and greater function.

Womb Breathing helps you free yourself from fear.

This method is from meditation science.

While sitting, you learn to breathe energy.

You do it to free yourself and feed

vital energy to the child in your womb.

You're made to breathe vital energy from the air.

You're made to feed vital energy to the child in your womb.

By sitting to calm and breathe in a deeper way

you can help your self and your child.

So please sit, as upright as possible, comfortable and at ease.

See that there's a luminous breathing vase

in the navel center in your energy body.

It's called the Vase of Life.

It's known and respected in different traditions.

Sense that you're made to breathe vital energy into the vase.

Sense that all your life you've been breathing energy in the air,

breathing it in and out without using it.

In order to breathe it in and down into the vase

you need to intend the energy in and down.

When you do you'll feel it go into the vase.

Now practice breathing energy from the air down into the vase.

As you continue to breathe energy into the Vase of Life

it absorbs up into your energy body channels.

Your child resonates with this energy,

becoming more alive.

Please do this sitting practice for at least twenty minutes in the morning.

Play the CD for audioguidance,

and then practice for a few minutes a few times a day.

Your body likes to do the practice.

You do Womb Breathing naturally.

The more you do it, the more it happens instinctively.

The more you practice, the more this breathing

will emerge spontaneously during labor.

Please do it now.

Breathe vital energy from the air into your Vase of Life.

Sit with effortless upright balance on the floor with cushions,

or sit in a chair if that's easier for you.

Sit upright into your body as if you're sitting into life itself.

Sit and breathe life into your vase for your child.

Shift your body a little if you need to.

Find your balance and breathe easily into your energy system.

Breathe with your belly and the Life Vase in your navel.

Sense the energy of the universal field all around you,

supporting you.

Breathe into it gently and deep.

Realize that you're made to use that energy to breathe in a greater way.

Engage the total sensation of your body,

your physical body and your energy body.

Feel yourself breathe completely.

Appreciate the many dimensions of life in you and your unborn child.

Breathe in a way that will give you and your child greater life.

Gain a sense of sacred body as you breathe in a deeper way.

With this breathing a child can be born free of fear.

Learn to breath-feed your energy system.

Allow yourself to absorb vital energy from the air.

Learn to breath-feed your child.

Breathe vital essence from the air.

You have a billionfold system of energy pathways.

You have a central energy channel with brilliant centers, alive with light.

You have an energy breathing vase in your navel center.

You have a body for a greater kind of birth.

You can give your child advantage, and life gain.

So please, sit and breathe in this way.

Breathe with open awareness.

Learn to sense the life-giving energy field all around you.

Breathe the energy of the universal life force.

Learn to support yourself in a greater way with what's available.

Know your energy body.

Breathe vital energy.

Breathe into the vase.

Breathe life into your vase for your child.

As you remain comfortably upright, breathing slow and deep,

notice when your mind distracts you.

You may find you're lost in thought,

no longer aware of breathing vital energy.

You lose that intention.

You may be thinking about something that happened,

or something that's going to happen.

You may be anxious about something and you're not present.

Then something wakes you up.

Your awareness wakes you up to breathe with intention.

Breathe universal energy, vital life-giving energy.

Slow down and go deep.

See how your mind may take you away,

and then your awareness wakes you up and brings you back.

Continue breathing vital energy.

Don't identify with thoughts that come up.

Don't identify with emotions.

Stay with energy breathing in bodily calm and open awareness.

Breathe energy easily.

Breathe into the vase.

Breathe life into the vase.

Feel the energy you breathe absorb into your body.

Feel the energy absorb into your child.

Feel how you both gain life.

During the practice, fears may arise in different ways,

causing anxious thoughts distracting you from being present.

It's important to recognize anxiety and fear.

Catch your fears and they tend to dissolve.

Return to awareness of energy breathing.

It's a matter of life.

Come to life.

Breathe life.

See that you can do this with ease.

Breathe into new function, with living awareness.

When you breathe this way, it helps you free yourself from thought.

It helps you free yourself from fear.

Breathe into your dynamic energy system.

Feel the energy gain.

The more you practice, the more you get it.

Be calm as thought and emotion come.

Breathe in open awareness.

Be undisturbed by thought.

Be undisturbed.

Continue energy breathing in open awareness.

Even when intense thoughts and emotions come,

you can keep calm.

You can be fearless when labor comes.

You can bring calm into childbirth.

Breathe energy in open awareness.

All of life, all the universe, is present here and now.

Come into presence more and more.

Breathe in living presence.

Do this practice to prepare for childbirth.

When labor comes, you can do this practice.

You can remain undisturbed.

Remain undisturbed.

This is the way to calm birth.

When a contraction comes, breathe it in.

See and dispel fears that arise.

As the contraction fades, return to energy breathing.

You're already doing it.

Relax and enjoy Womb Breathing.

It helps you stay calm in contractions.

Breathe calm between contractions.

Rest and breathe in awareness.

Breathe free.

This is a path of life.

This is the breath of life,

all the life energy and oxygen you need.

You're more alive in your breathing.

You're enjoying greater function.

Do something important for your child.

Do something important for your self.

Continue breathing into the vase.

Calm Birth Practice Three: Giving and Receiving

Giving and Receiving is a famous healing practice from ancient wisdom applied to childbirth. The intention is that women will discover natural healing ability in themselves in preparing to give birth. This can help them heal anything that may need to be healed in themselves. It may also remind the women that they have a gift and more potential than they imagined. It's a practice of empathic breathing, compassionate breathing.

The availability of the practice and the challenges of medical birth are incentives for pregnant women to practice healing, to try to give birth to a healthier generation.

Giving and Receiving enables women to spontaneously come into new relationship with their body to practice the healing of their own birth experience.

Pregnant women are able to practice the healing of conditions that may be present in themselves or in the unborn child. The women are able to calm the wombchild from disturbances that may come in from conception onward, to prevent any such disturbances from affecting child development. Giving and Receiving is a method for dual maternal-fetal healing.

Giving and Receiving may be used as a method of labor pain management. Like Womb Breathing, it can help women use the experience of labor to empower themselves.

This ancient wisdom method has been called "The Holy Secret" and "The Wish-Fulfilling Gem." Compassion is the wish-fulfilling gem. It's a Buddhist practice in use in the medical field today. It's called *ton len* in Tibetan, which has been translated as "sending and receiving" or "exchanging oneself for another." It's a direct healing method that can be used to decrease anxiety and suffering and to reverse harmful conditions. Giving and Receiving helps women use inherent healing skills to redefine childbirth. The practice adds to a woman's empowerment potential in the childbirth process.

The basis of the practice is twofold: inherent compassion capability and the radiant energetic nature of the human body. The energy body is the basis of inborn healing potential.

People on the birth team can do this practice to help the woman and child. They breathe in, taking to heart the energy of pain or stress that the woman and child may have, taking it into body light. It's in their nature that they can breathe out radiant healing energy into the woman and child. If the birth is premature or for any problem the woman or child may have, anyone connected to the birth can participate by practicing healing them both with Giving and Receiving. Don't doubt that it can have an effect.

The more time spent engaged in this practice, the more effective it will probably be. As the pregnant woman practices healing herself and her child, entering her unlimited nature, she brings the practice and experience of healing into birth.

Key Points

» In this practice, women connect with their innate healing ability, and they open to another dimension of healthy activity in childbirth.

» It's healing to practice healing. The intention to heal one's self or another tends to raise healing energy in the person who intends. Practicing healing may be vital to childbirth health.

» The use of Giving and Receiving throughout prenatal care can develop women's ability to take in pain without taking it on in labor.

» With this practice, women may experience a new sense of body and ability in preparing to give birth.

» Most women can do this with proper instruction.

The Method

Giving and Receiving can be practiced in any posture, at any time, but it's most effective to do this practice sitting. A pregnant woman can practice Giving and Receiving for herself or for the child, or for both simultaneously. In this program, it's used for prenatal care, for labor and delivery, and for postnatal care.

Please note that Giving and Receiving differs importantly from Womb Breathing. With Womb Breathing, a woman breathes vital energy from the air into her energy body. The exhale is simple release. With Giving and Receiving, she compassionately takes in the energy of the suffering of someone, herself or another, and she sees that energy dissolve into natural light in her body. She breathes out healing energy into herself, her child, or someone else. With Giving and Receiving, the woman not only breathes into her energy body, she breathes out of her energy body, exhaling and radiating out energies that can be received far away. *Womb Breathing and Giving and Receiving must be practiced separately.*

A woman can prepare for conception and childbirth by practicing healing anything in herself that might need to be healed. That could include the energy of any trauma and / or shock that may remain from her own birth. She can sit and follow the natural flow of her breath, easily and deeply. On her inhale, she can breathe in, take in, the energy of any remaining traces of her birth shock or trauma. What is breathed in, empathically taken in, dissolves into natural light in her body. She can breathe out into herself abundant healing energy. The breathing is not forced in any way. It can be effortless.

The breaths can be gentle and short, or longer and fuller, as long as it's in the natural flow of the breath. The transition from inhale to exhale is effortless. What the woman takes in is brought in with compassion. It is taken to heart and dissolves into light in her body. The giving out of healing energy is bountiful, given freely and graciously, generously, because the woman has found her unlimited life.

To do the practice for her child, the woman breathes in and takes to heart the energy of any difficulty that the child may have, however subtle it may be. She sees that energy dissolve into light in her body, and she breathes out healing energy into the child. What she intentionally takes in dissolves into live light in her energy body, and she effortlessly breathes out the energy of healing intention into the child in her womb.

Breathing into Contractions

A woman practicing Giving and Receiving during labor contractions inhales the pain of the contraction right into light in her body, and she sends healing energy into the child being squeezed in her womb. Her partner may also do this with her, for her and the child, breathing healing energy into birth.

Giving and Receiving can be an inspired way to use both the inhale and the exhale in labor contractions. Breathing in, the woman accepts the intensity, and compassionately takes it in. Breathing out, she sends healing intention into herself and the child at the same time as releasing pain and stress.

Breathing into contractions as early as possible in labor enables women to gain psychological strength progressively throughout contractions, to recognize and dispel anxieties that may arise.

If a woman can practice Giving and Receiving to ride through contractions, she probably will have a very good experience giving birth, and her baby will probably have a very good birthday.

The Practice (the audioguide, line by line)

Giving and Receiving is a famous practice from ancient wisdom applied to childbirth.

It's the practice of breathing healing.

It can bring healing into childbirth.

It's for whatever may need to be healed in the pregnant woman, her partner, or the child in the womb.

Sitting upright, balanced, at ease,

go with the natural flow of your breath.

Breathe in any health problems you may have.

Let the condition or disturbance dissolve in light in your body.

Breathe out into your self the healing energy you need.

Please practice this method of breathing.

On the in-breath, take in any disturbances there may be

in you, or in your child. Take that to heart.

See it dissolve in light in your body.

With the out-breath, intend healing energies

into yourself, or into the child, or into you both.

A child who is well

receives the energy as blessings.

Practice Giving and Receiving often.

Please do it now.

In the natural flow of your breath,

breathe in any difficulty that may be in you or in your child.

Take it to heart.

See that energy dissolve into light in your body,

and breathe out into your self and your child

all the healing energy you may need.

Breathe, healing yourself and your child.

Practice compassionate healing with your breath.

Compassionate breathing is empowering and far-reaching.

You can breathe back into your own birth experience.

Any disturbance that may remain from then

may be released by this practice now,

helping your child to be free.

What you breathe in from your birth dissolves in natural light in you.

Breathe out into your self and your child

all the healing energy you both may need.

It's time to heal with the breath.

Now turning towards another pregnant woman, someone in distress,

breathe into your body light any disturbance she may have.

You can do this easily, just as you did for yourself and your child.

Whatever you breathe in dissolves in your living light.

Effortlessly breathe out into that pregnant woman

all the healing energy she may need.

Please practice healing now.

There's no separation in the universal field.

You can reach any person directly in yourself,

wherever they are.

As you breathe in another woman's health challenges

you inseparably breathe in your own.

Breathe in easily, effortlessly giving that woman

your compassionate care.

All that you take in dissolves in light in you.

Breathe out, sending energies that nourish and heal.

Trust your ability to heal.

Now please turn your attention to two or three anxious pregnant women.

Effortlessly breathe their challenges into living light in you.

Intend calming healing energy into those women.

Extend this practice of compassionate breathing now.

Please do it.

Taking this practice to a larger number of people,

think of a birthing center you know.

Imagine all the pregnant women, their partners,

the birthing personnel.

Go beyond what you think you can do.

Breathe in their stresses and intensity.

Let it all dissolve in the light in your body.

With clear intention, breathe out calming healing energy

into all the people in the birthing center at once.

Give grace to the birthing center now.

You can do this.

When your labor contractions start,

you can breathe in the contraction.

You can breathe out opening.

If you practice now

you can prevent yourself from suffering.

You can breathe in the contraction.

You can breathe out release.

You can breathe grace into labor.

Please practice that now.

This is an ancient practice

proven effective through centuries of use.

Giving and Receiving can be done anywhere, anytime.

Be fearless in doing this compassionate breathing.

See that what you take in dissolves in light in you.

What you send out instantly connects.

The more you do this practice for yourself and your child,

the more effective it becomes.

The more you do this practice for others,

the more you heal your self and your child.

The more you do this practice, the more life-giving you become.

This practice can be vital in postnatal care.

Please do this practice often.

VI
Calm Births

Birth stories told by women who were active participants in giving birth often express a good deal of practical wisdom, inspiration, and informa- tion for other women. Positive stories shared by women who have had wonderful childbirth experiences are an irreplaceable way to transmit knowledge of a woman's true capacities in pregnancy and birth.

—Ina May Gaskin[74]

Following is a selection of interviews and reports written by women who have given birth using the Calm Birth practice. The reports are postnatal unless otherwise indicated. It is documentation of applied prenatal meditation spanning seventeen years. They are descriptions of women's experiences of new childbirth practice.

Logan Jaymes

Baby: Logan Jaymes
Parents: Ana and Chris
Birth date: 7/6/15
Birth weight: 8 lb.

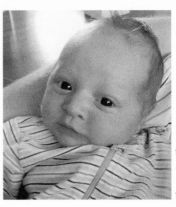

Photos by Chris Jorgensen

After their first birth transferred from home to hospital and ended in a cesarean, Ana and Chris knew that they wanted to approach the next pregnancy with a new kind of preparation.

Ana: We wanted to give the baby the best that we could, something that he could feel that he was being birthed with love and not stress. I wanted to be totally aware, and for him to be aware. I wanted to not feel afraid … I just wanted the baby to be healthy, and just to give the best to my baby, the best slow and gentle and loving birth.

A family friend told Ana and Chris about Anna H., a doula who teaches Calm Birth (and also conducted this interview), and they started taking her classes at the end of the pregnancy.

Ana: Because I took Hypnobirthing before and it didn't really work for me, I was open-minded to listen to something new, but I knew that in the end I would make the decision of what I wanted to do. In Hypnobirthing, I said, "This is what I have to do," and it was stressful for me. This time, I said that I would listen to what Calm Birth had to say, but at the end, I knew that I could do whatever I wanted, and if it didn't work for me, I'd do what did work for me. It felt really comforting to know that it was my decision, and that I didn't have any pressure to follow any method—it was just listening to different ideas, knowing that once I was in labor, I'd know what to do. The CD helped me to remember to breathe, and that I needed to take things slow and relax and keep focus so that labor could go smoothly.

Chris joined Ana in practicing the CD. "I understand the importance of meditation and calming and relaxing your body," he says, "So it was enjoyable to set time aside to do it."

Labor started on the Fourth of July. Ana, Chris, and their eighteen-month-old son, Sebastian, went to the parade while Ana breathed through early labor contractions. She called Anna H., her doula, around three in the morning. For the next nineteen hours, Ana labored at home, attended by Chris and Anna H. They went for walks, ate, and listened to Practice of Opening and Womb Breathing from time to time, when Ana wanted to rest or center with her breathing. Around 7 pm, Ana was experiencing very regular contractions, and around 10 pm they called the hospital birth center.

Due to unforeseen and unusual circumstances, the only birth center in the valley that supported vaginal births after cesarean (VBACs) was closed, and Ana's doctor was unreachable when Anna H. called.

Anna H.: This was one of the most intense experiences I've had as a doula. I found that I was really focusing on my breathing to keep me centered. The thought that we would have to go someplace where you might not feel supported by the staff to deliver and make your choices.... Something we talk about a lot in Calm Birth is being able to recognize and release fears as they came up, and I found myself doing a lot of that.

Ana: I thought, "If I'm not gonna be able to go where I'd planned, I'm obviously going to have a C-section." And then I thought, "Well, then I don't wanna feel any more contractions if I'm just gonna have a cesarean," so I got in the shower because I thought that would stop the contractions and it did, for a little bit, and I told Chris and Anna to figure it out. I was really focused on my contractions and what I was doing. If I lost control, I would feel pain, and I didn't want to focus on it or fixate on it; if we were going to go have a

C-section, I thought we should just do it ... but I also felt like it was everything for nothing. I did everything, and we'd been there all day, and we'd been doing so great, and we were ready to go, and now I was just going to go have a C-section, like it was all for nothing? I felt kind of disappointed, but I believe in prayer, and I'd prayed about it before and asked Heavenly Father if I would have a natural birth and the answer was yes. So it reminded me that something was going to work out, because I believe in those answers, and that calmed me down. I just needed to wait to see what would happen, and everything got figured out.

Breathing has a lot to do with staying focused and losing stress, and not tensing up. Especially during labor, if I tense, I felt pain, and when I was focusing and breathing calmly, there was no pain! I mean, a little bit, but not really. And that's why I wanted to keep focusing and do my thing and relax, and I knew something would work out.

Anna H.: And it did! You seemed to really keep your center in the face of all that intensity. We got ahold of your doctor and arranged to meet at the other hospital.

Ana: I was happy that I would still be able to have my natural birth, and I think that kept me happy and with my hopes up. We drove to the hospital, walked in, went straight to the room, and the nurse checked me and said I was at 8. Right after she checked, the water broke, and I was very happy about that—I didn't want it to break artificially. Then I was at 9½. My body started pushing, and the nurses said, "Don't push!" and I couldn't help it, my body was doing it. Right after that, they checked again and I was at 10, and the doctor got there. Then we were able to continue with the birth, and it wasn't long after that that he was born!

Anna H.: How did it compare to the postpartum meeting with Sebastian?

Ana: It was huge! When I had my first son, and they took him out with a C-section, I was so medicated that I wanted to hold him so much, but I couldn't keep my eyes open, and that felt really sad. I didn't like them taking him away from me so fast and not being able to hold him right away. It was so sad for me, and this time, him [Logan] being placed on my stomach right away, combined with the whole feeling of "I did it! I did it, and it wasn't as bad as I thought it would be, and I could do it again, and I got to do everything I wanted—for the most part." I gave my son a natural birth without meds, as gentle as we could, and he didn't get stressed, and that made me feel really, really happy.

Anna H.: How's the postpartum period been?

Ana: Amazing. After Sebastian was born, I was depressed for months and months. And I wasn't sleeping well, obviously, but with the depression everything was worse. I didn't want to go out, I didn't want to shower or do my hair, I would just cry and talk to my son all day, and having a cesarean I felt like I couldn't do anything—I couldn't clean the house; it just made things worse.

This time, after a vaginal birth, I felt normal, like I could do whatever I wanted! I had to remind myself to take it easy. After a vaginal birth, you feel normal, not like you're cut open, and you just feel so powerful and happy! The next day, when we were in the hospital, I had a huge smile! I was saying to all the nurses, "How are you? I'm great! I had a vaginal birth. I'm so happy!" and when we walked out of the hospital, I was smiling… it was a huge difference. I feel so so happy!

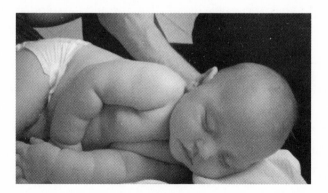

Anna H.: I know you prayed a lot about this and did massage and prenatal yoga, but how do you feel like Calm Birth specifically contributed to your overall experience?

Ana: I honestly think that breathing has a lot to do with not feeling stress. It has to do with keeping your blood pressure down! These days, the way birth is, it's like, "You have forty-two weeks or we're gonna induce or take the baby out," it makes people stressed! It makes mamas stressed, and I've seen a lot of pregnant women whose blood pressure goes up, and they have to be induced because of it and they end up having an epidural or cesarean, and it's really sad! And I think that breathing can keep all those things away! When you're feeling stressed, especially when you want to avoid a cesarean and you only have an amount of time to go into labor, and there are so many things that you just... you're a little bit stressed! And breathing can really help keep you calm, and your blood pressure down. I learned that a lot. Also, during labor, if I didn't do calm breathing the way I'd learned, I felt pain. And when I did it correctly: no pain!

Anna H.: So, when you say no pain, I'm assuming you were still having sensation?

Ana: Yeah, absolutely. But it was like, "Okay, I know what it feels like, and I know it's uncomfortable, but if I breathe like this I can handle it, and it will go away, three minutes later it's gonna happen again," but definitely I know that if I wasn't breathing correctly I wouldn't have been able to handle it; I would have ended up in the hospital asking for pain medication or something like that.

Anna H.: Chris, how did you deal with that stress?

Chris: More than anything, what I've always tried to do is remain as calm as possible because I think clearer, and stressing out doesn't help anything. I've done lots of meditation and stuff before, so it was nice to be able to take a step back, ask what we could do, and how to keep as much to our birth plan as possible, to keep the big picture and stand our ground—but stay headstrong within reason, direct on our wishes.

Anna H.: Now, you two are pretty spiritual/religious people, of the Mormon faith. Did you feel like Calm Birth was harmonious with that?

Ana: Yes. With religion, it always has to do with remaining calm so you can think clearly and make good decisions. And when you are calm—which Calm Birth's breathing helps you remain calm—you can treat people nicely, have better relationships, live more clearly. If you're stressed, not-good things happen. Calm breathing helps you stay relaxed.

Chris: What we were taught is that meditation and prayer are the same thing; you're finding peace with yourself whether it's you and the Universe or you and a God above; realizing that you can't do everything yourself, that you're so small in the scheme of things, but that through meditation and prayer, you're able to get through hard things and remain calm because of it. Calm Birth helps us realize the importance of doing a daily meditation or prayer.

Anna H.: Do you feel like you'll continue to use these methods you've used?

Ana: Yes! Parenting can be really stressful. Having little ones and trying to give them the best and to have patience, to talk to them nicely when they're screaming at you, or when they all need something at the same time, breathing the way Calm Birth teaches really helps you have patience and be nice to your kids. Even when you're tired and having a hard time, you can just stop and remember and breathe; you can talk to them in a different way. If you don't, you can get stressed and yell at them, and then you feel bad because of that! I use calm breathing all the time. When I was pregnant, I practiced it to a point that that was how I wanted to breathe all the time, not just during pregnancy and not just during birth, because I'm more calm, more relaxed, and healthier! I feel like I have more air coming into my body. I realized how different I was breathing before, how shallow and how I wasn't getting enough air. Now I don't think about breathing like this ... when I stop and think about it, I always realize that I am breathing like this.

I think anyone could benefit from this. I mean, if you think about it, the littlest thing like breathing can change a lot! One of my cousins does a lot of meditation, and he said, "Have you noticed how babies breathe? And that we don't breathe the same way, and that we should?" And I didn't practice it, and I didn't think about it, until this class! And if you think about it, we come to this planet knowing how to breathe, but then we grow older and we switch it ... things happen, and we start breathing differently, and whether we see it or not, it has a huge impact in our bodies, in our selves! It's wonderful to see how something so little can change so much.

Julius Rawson

Baby: Julius Rawson
Parents: Rachael and Jeff
Birth date: 7/1/13
Birth weight: 8 lb. 6 oz.

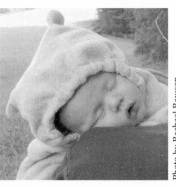

Photo by Rachael Rawson

Rachael: "Our son was born on July 1, 2013, and is now two years old. What a journey! As I write this, we're living in a small town in southwest Germany. I am four months pregnant with our second child, and have just pulled out my old Calm Birth CD to begin practicing again.

I took my doula's Calm Birth course about one month before my due date. Perhaps because I took the course so late in the pregnancy, I was quite dedicated to practicing on a daily basis until the birth. I enjoyed reading the textbook and getting to know the three meditations. My favorite, which I listened to almost exclusively for the last several weeks, was Womb Breathing. As I was laboring at the hospital, my husband or doula made sure the track was playing at all times. Our instructor also suggested that keeping a notebook of the practice might help encourage us to keep up with the meditations; I don't think I started that immediately, but kept daily notes for the last few weeks. On each day, I noted which meditation(s) I listened to, which foot was tucked in closer as I sat cross-legged (trying not to favor my favorite side), observations about each session, and any notable responses from the baby. A few examples:

Sun. 6/16: Womb Breathing; 7:30 am (Left foot in)
     Body a bit twitchy. Mind felt calm. 20 min flew by.
     Baby's responses: fair amount of movement. Responded when I intended energy to baby.

Wed. 6/19: WB; 7:10 am (Right foot in)
     A bit noisy mind today, distracted. Baby moved early on, and again toward end.

Sat. 6/22: WB; 7:15 am (R ft in)
     Fairly calm throughout. Not w/o mental chatter. Breathing helped wake me up today.
     Baby: some undulations, esp. toward end.

Fri. 6/28: WB; 7:25 am (R ft in)
     Distracted first half, relaxed into it. Worry about date for inducement (July 11) if labor is late in coming. Let it go....
     Baby: subtle while sitting.

Sat. 6/29: WB; 7:50 am (L ft in)
     Very similar to past few days. Body comfortable, mind prone to wandering, worrying. Settles somewhat over course.
     Baby: fairly still, tight uterus (Braxton Hicks). a little mvt. @ end.

Sun. 6/30: WB; 7:30 am (R ft in)

Imagining labor coming on.

Baby napping ☺

Mon. 7/1: WB; 7:15 am (L ft in)

A bit crampy. Water broke or cervical plug? Clear discharge, slightly pinkish, wet pad. Did Practice of Opening.

Baby: some movement, also uterine and low back minor cramping.

The last entry is a bit graphic, but it was quite a powerful moment, and in hindsight, was the beginning of my labor! I began my meditation as usual, and felt a little wetness, which I assumed was a bit of escaped urine, since by this point I had to pee all the time. I finished the meditation and went to the toilet and discovered the discharge was pink in color, which started a series of speculations, leading to us calling the doctor around 8 am. She thought it might indicate the start of labor, but that we would have a lot of time ahead of us. Within an hour or so, the contractions were coming closer, at a much faster rate than we were led to expect in the birthing class, and our birthing day "plan" of watching movies, playing games, etc., to fill in the space of the long day and night ahead started to seem improbable.

When I suggested to my husband at 9:30 or 10 am that we start the movie we'd picked out, he thought I was crazy! The contractions seemed frequent and intense enough that we went to the hospital around 11 am and were admitted shortly thereafter. Throughout the labor, our CD player was looping Track 2, Womb Breathing. I was very lucky to have had a baby who was healthy, ready, and came relatively easily and quickly. He was born just after 4 pm that afternoon. I didn't feel that I had to endure any excruciating pain, and was happy to avoid the need for drugs to dull the intensity of the contractions. My husband had also practiced some of the acupressure points recommended for labor contractions (among lots of information provided by my doula!), and having him press hard on the lower-back points during the intense moments of the contractions was a huge comfort throughout the labor.

It's hard to quantify precisely how my labor was impacted by my practice and use of the Calm Birth meditations, but I can say with confidence that meditating on a daily, or occasionally twice daily, basis for over a month was the single most consistent meditation routine I have ever practiced, before or since giving birth. The meditations became very familiar, but different words, images, or phrases would come into focus on different days. The affirmations of the meditations themselves gave me a sense of calm and confidence that I was ready and prepared to labor, even though it was a fully new and unknown experience to me. I don't think any amount of meditation or birthing education can actually direct one's labor to achieve a particular desired outcome, but I believe that having a familiar and calming routine to bring one's mind back to the present and back to the breath is extremely useful throughout the labor. It is an intense and out-of-body experience, and a time when the mind can easily get overwhelmed with the emotions, physicality, and extended timespan of the labor. I feel the effort spent on this mental preparation for birth was well worth every minute.

Emilis

Baby: Emilis
Parents: Dovile and Thomas
Birth date: 4/7/13
Birth weight: 8 lb. 2 oz.

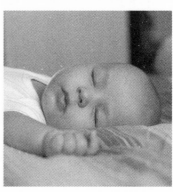

Photo by Dovilė Karvauskienė

Dovile was twenty-three years old and had studied and practiced meditation for years with her husband. They lived in Lithuania. After Dovile became pregnant, she went online to find a childbirth method using meditation. She couldn't find anything like that in Lithuania or in Russia. Then she came upon the Calm Birth website and saw the images of pregnant women meditating. She contacted the Calm Birth office and asked to be trained in childbirth meditation for her own birth, and then to establish the program in Lithuania.

Dovile: I gave birth on April 7. Now I am very grateful for this method because my birth would not have been as quick, conscious, and fearless as it was. I was doing Womb Breathing all the time at home. I knew the whole CD by heart. While meditating to prepare for the birth, my fears kept coming up.

I concentrated on recognizing fear. And then there was no fear on my birth day! I was cheerful all the time. The doctors even thought that nothing was happening to me because apparently this was very unusual for them. I was doing Womb Breathing during every contraction. When we came to hospital, I was 5 cm dilated (almost without pain), and after about two hours I was fully dilated. The contractions were painful but bearable. I didn't use any drugs or painkillers. Everything was natural.

Womb Breathing helped me to be conscious, so that's why I was telling myself to stay relaxed, to not concentrate on pain. I'm sure that all this wouldn't have happened without Womb Breathing.

Hana Leigh

Baby: Hana Leigh
Parents: Clee and Austen
Birth date: 2/26/01
Birth weight: 7 lb. 4 oz.

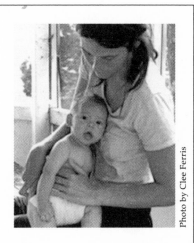

Photo by Clee Ferris

Late in her third pregnancy, Clee expressed interest in meditation to a midwife she had just chosen to help her with her birth, which she wanted to be completely natural. The midwife had heard of Calm Birth and recommended that Clee get in touch with the program. The result was that even though Clee received the Womb Breathing and Practice of Opening instructions only eight days before the birth, the following account testifies that even if a woman is introduced to Calm Birth meditation toward the end of the pregnancy, the practice can be transformative.

CB (Whitney Wolf, interviewer): Hana Leigh was born eight days after you were introduced to the Calm Birth methods. What were your first experiences, once you received the Calm Birth instructions?

Clee: Just taking the time to sit, to be centered, and go inward, and to check in. That quiet space. It really helped a lot.

CB: How did you find taking that inward space helpful at that point in your pregnancy?

Clee: It helped to reduce stress and clarify some things within myself. It provided me a calm space. It definitely helped me to calm down and feel more centered and balanced, and ready to deal with the next day, with my other children, and all the input and stimulation of the day.

CB: How would you describe your experience of the meditation?

Clee: Definitely a sense of being more centered, calm, and present. I was able to stay that way even with a lot of things that were going on. During the birth, I was able to be in the present moment, with the pain, not wondering what it would be in an hour from now, or going away from the moment. It really helped me to be fully in the birth experience.

CB: Austen, did you have any kind of experience where you could imagine the womb in yourself with the child in your womb?

Austen: Yes, definitely. I had a couple of dreams that were very lucid where I felt that I was pregnant and I could feel Hana Leigh was really active in my belly. She was moving around. Actually, I think what happened is that I fell asleep with my hand on Clee's belly and she was moving all around when I fell into a dream space with that happening. And then I had this dream that she was in my tummy moving all around and I think that in the real space my hand was still on Clee's belly. I remember doing the breath meditation and I felt a sense of warm energy in my tummy. The sense of breathing to nourish your baby felt really good and I could connect with that. The Womb Breathing actually helped me to remember to breathe to nourish my own inner baby. It was great.

Clee: Yes, it was nice to share that experience together.

CB: By having the Calm Birth meditation, how did this pregnancy differ from your previous pregnancies?

Clee: This time in the actual labor I was able to be more in the moment, breathing and opening up to that pain, not resisting it as I had done before. I attribute that to a lot of things, but it helped me by listening to the CD and practicing, being more aware and in the moment and more able to open up to that pain rather than resisting it.

CB: How did the meditation help you with the pain?

Clee: Being present with the pain and not resisting it was amazing. It was the most powerful, wonderful experience. It was a journey and a great adventure rather than a scary, drawn-out nightmare.

CB: The pain and the fear appear to be connected. If you resist the pain, it leads to more fear. If you surrender and open, the fear and resistance seem to resolve themselves.

Clee: Exactly. Because being in the moment, you are just being there, fully feeling. You are open and just there. Fear for me comes when you're worrying what is going to happen, the next contraction, or when the baby comes, grasping for a moment that isn't real. Then you are missing out on being in the moment, not being able to be open, because you are resisting something that has not even happened. It is kind of hard to explain. I would say that the pain didn't feel as painful because the breathing meditation stayed with me.

CB: Austen, as soon as Clee brought the CD home, you started practicing with her. How did that affect you?

Austen: It definitely helped me with a sense of connection. It helped shift me into a balanced perspective. Whereas before, being a father in a pregnancy you are feeling a sense of more like "I am going to take care of the other duties. I am not really in charge of nourishing the baby in the body besides cooking meals for the mama." It reminded me, it might have been something that I read or heard on the Calm Birth CD, that the father is important, spiritually and energetically nourishing the baby with his thoughts and energy. So there is a real connection. It definitely helped me to see that... After receiving the meditation and before she was born, it was really rich with magical experiences. Probably dreams too, but it's hard to remember.

Clee: That's because it was like a kind of dreamy space around the birth.

Austen: We talked about it being only eight days that we had the CD, but when Clee first heard from Rhione, the midwife, about this opportunity, that someone was writing a book and was offering classes and the CD, that was sort of like the initial connection. That was the first time I'd really heard of anything about pregnant women or couples meditating to alleviate the fears and discomforts in labor. I'd never heard anything about that. That was a couple of weeks prior to when Clee met you and received the practices.

Clee: The day before the birth, I came outside and hung out. We had a beautiful, wonderful day. I was having light cramping. Went to bed that night and woke up about three in the morning. What I recall is Anaya [their two-year-old son] screaming "baby" in the middle of the night and waking me up. That is what I recall. I recall him saying "BABY," and I was in labor! It was pretty amazing. And I woke up and said, "I'm in labor." ... Then I said that I was cold, so we made the house really warm. I asked Austen to time the contractions. I thought the baby was going to come relatively quickly. So, I was really able to be present, to really open up to the pain.

CB: I know that when we first met, when we first instructed you in the practice, you shared with me that you wanted to really come to a place where you could open and surrender.

Clee: That was my big hope for my experience with labor, and I was really able to do that, and it was so great. I was able to go through labor by myself for a while, until the midwives arrived. They got here just as the sun was rising.

Austen: They got here right when the light was coming in. It was amazing. They had just walked in. We had had some worries that Anaya and Kai' [their sons] would be upset and be awake and want lots of attention. But they were sound asleep, and they slept through the majority of it.

Clee: Anaya woke up about an hour before the birth... I went on amazing journeys. I just went into myself and it was like I was feeling myself like you were talking about in the meditation CD, how you can get way out there and the voice brings me back; I was able to bring myself back. I would get real involved in the pain and then I would feel okay. Then I would imagine whales under water giving birth, and I would think, wow, you know, I can do this. And then I thought about all of the women who were giving birth in that moment and all those who have given birth. I was really able to ground myself in these real feelings of power and the beauty of it, rather than feeling I can't do this because it's such a hard thing. "I am doing this! There are hundreds of women doing this right now. I can do this! I am doing it!"... The midwives came in, and we were sitting there. I was able to let them touch my body and open up to their love, and the same with Austen, without feeling resistance. Then the contractions started getting really strong and the pain was getting more and more difficult for me to handle. I said that I wanted to get into the water and I did. Not too long after I got in the water, maybe an hour, she was born.

Austen: Just as the sun was rising—I remember them saying, "Oh, I see her head," and I was holding Anaya and walking around. Maybe it was ten minutes before she was born that the sun peeked—there is a ridge on the east side, and there was this glimmer of sun peeking over that ridge.

Clee: I was really calm. I remembered that in my last two childbirths, the pushing part in the last intense part of labor was like screaming for me. This time I was able to use my voice and make these real guttural songs. [She expressed her sound.]

Austen: Yes. I've heard these sounds in songs before in Tibetan chants sung by monks that are real deep. That's what she sounded like when she was in the water.

Clee: It was awesome.

CB: Have you ever experienced these sounds in yourself before?

Clee: Not in myself. No. It felt so good. I felt so grounded and rooted in strength, like, ah—the earth. I really don't have words for it, but it really helped me. It was a tool for using my voice like I had been wanting to do in my previous births, without screaming or distress.

CB: Were you aware of your breathing during the contractions, or in delivery, by returning to Womb Breathing?

Clee: Oh yes. I was very conscious of my breath throughout, the whole way. While I was going on a journey inside myself, the breath was the physical manifestation of the other part that was helping me remain open, helping me to be flexible and open. It was the breath.

CB: When the contractions relaxed, did you find yourself doing the Womb Breathing?

Clee: Yes. Right in between while I was awaiting the next contraction and I was taking time to breathe and center myself.

Austen: And she was subconsciously doing Womb Breathing. Her body reverted to that naturally.

Clee: Definitely. Yes. It was really great. It was beautiful. It was wonderful. It went really smoothly. It was really calm. Hana Leigh came out, and she was just sitting there and I rubbed her back and it was a really peaceful space for her to come into. Everything had been peaceful.

Austen: The midwives commented that it was hard for them to leave this house.

CB: How was it hard for them to leave?

Austen: Because it was being in life itself. Sometimes, you know, the labor gets intense and people are all involved and there is lots of tension and the woman is in a lot of pain rather than letting it just flow. Clee was really able to handle the intensity of energy [Clee comments with "Yes"], to be able to handle it and harness it rather than fight it, because it is literally like the universe pouring through the mother giving birth. That energy is coming through. Clee let the energy flow rather than be afraid of it. At one point one of the midwives commented that she has been doing childbirth for a long time and it was a great day for other women across the world giving birth, because they could tap into that energy that Clee was experiencing.

Clee: Every step of the way, the first thing I would do was check in with her [Hana Leigh] and recognize that this pain is bringing my baby closer to me. I don't know other than I was just opening up to her coming through. It was like I was in a process of birth. I felt like that is how I had to prepare myself to be her mother and to know her.

CB: Was there a need to push?

Clee: I did go through a little bit of wanting to bear down and push as hard as I could, and I did that: push, push, push. It was really hard. Then the attending midwives reminded me, saying, "Open yourself up and allow the baby to come through and be with your breath." Then I was able to let her come through more naturally rather than trying to push. I experienced both sides of what you are saying: feeling the desire to get the pain over with, and the releasing through my breath.

CB: What do you feel was the urge to want to push?

Clee: I was ready for her to come out. "I want to see you now. You're so close." And then wanting to be in control of it, wanting to be active in it rather than opening up and being responsible with this energy.

CB: Impatient with the timing—

Austen: Yeah, wanting to have a sense of control.

CB: What was the difference when you were pushing versus when you felt that you were being moved?

Clee: When I was trying to push, there was a sense of forceful energy trying to get something out. She was resisting it.

CB: How did you know that?

Clee: It was a feeling that she would come down and slip back up and I could feel her doing it. There was a sense of trying to make something happen while not really knowing if it's not going to happen. If you just keep pushing, pushing, pushing, pushing, it's resistance.

CB: Would you say that the Calm Birth meditation was helpful for you to listen to your instincts?

Clee: Yes, definitely. I can imagine had I implemented it much earlier, it could have been even more helpful. Taking the time to do that for myself, to listen to the CD and do the practice. That's a key. I think women would really benefit from that, taking the time and space to breathe and go within.

CB: Do you feel that you accomplished what your intention was when we first met when you expressed to me what your concerns were and what you wanted to accomplish with this labor and delivery with Hana Leigh?

Clee: Oh yes. I was definitely able to do what I wanted to, which was to open up and allow the universe of life to be poured through me and be able to embrace it and enjoy it and see it as a real gift. When you fully open up to it, it's this amazing, strong, powerful love flowing through you! It's really an amazing gift!

CB: I can feel it right now with you voicing it; the power went right through me, the power again, how beautiful.

Clee: It is and I feel blessed to have been able to get to a space to feel it, instead of resisting it and being afraid of it, because it is really powerful.

Lucy

Baby: Lucy Capri
Parents: Nell and Charles
Birth date: 6/21/09
Birth weight: 6 lb. 5.2 oz.

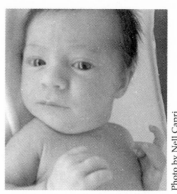

Photo by Nell Capri

Nell: The practice of Calm Birth gave our daughter a peaceful beginning. Not only did Calm Birth help us on the day of her birth, but also during my pregnancy and the days following delivery. It has become a way of life for us. I was a few days overdue and, to my frustration, an induction was planned. More than anything, I wanted to have a natural birth; and while I knew certain variables were out of my hands, with what I had learned I knew I could control how I handled the situation we were in. Adrienne, our instructor, helped my husband and me feel that we had the power and control over what our delivery could be, and that even if I ended up having to be induced, with what we learned in Calm Birth we could still have a peaceful birth.

On Saturday evening, I noticed I was having a little more discomfort, but didn't think much of it. After all, we were forty weeks and change … it was going to be a bit uncomfortable. Around 4 am, what I thought were my Braxton Hicks contractions were coming at about four to five minutes apart. I was too uncomfortable to be in bed, so I made my way to the kitchen to clean. It never occurred to me that I was actually in labor! I was excited to finally have some Braxton Hicks to which I could practice my breathing. Never once did I feel concerned or alarmed. I always felt at peace. Around 6:30 am, I had a pretty big contraction in my bedroom. During my contraction, my husband Charles woke up and said, "You're in labor!" I thought they were still Braxton Hicks and four to five minutes apart. To entertain him, we timed my contractions and realized they were one to two minutes apart lasting about one minute each. The intensity of the contractions really sent me to the floor, but I just used my Womb Breathing and felt good.

At this point, I thought, "Okay, maybe this is the real thing," so I let Charles call the doctor. I did reemphasize to him that I was not going until I had to, not wanting to be tied down to a hospital bed for hours on end. Knowing that the time to go was drawing near, I made my way to the shower. I took my sweet time, enjoying the hot water, doing my Womb Breathing through the contractions while singing Jimmy Buffett. I have to reiterate how in control, natural, and at peace I felt. We made our way to the hospital, and upon our arrival, the contractions were really getting intense. I was concentrating more, and the Womb Breathing helped me find a rhythm and stay in my zone.

I was checked into the OB ward and to my relief found out that I was not a pansy, that the contractions were real and not Braxton Hicks. I was 9 cm dilated with my bag of waters bulging! I walked to the labor room and was asked to get into bed. The philosophy of Calm Birth really helped my husband and me at this stage. We were now in unfamiliar territory, and the birth was upon us. This is when we really needed to rely on each other and what we had learned, to stay calm and positive. We made the room a comfortable environment by dimming the lights and putting on Jimmy Buffett and Reckless Kelly. When the time came to have Lucy, I thought I'd want some more relaxing music or my Calm Birth CD, but I really wanted to listen to Jimmy Buffett and do my Womb Breathing to that!

After an hour of intense pushing on my back, I was getting tired and flustered. I really wanted to use the other positions that Adrienne had taught me, but I was scared to ask. Luckily, Charles read my mind and asked for me. Our doctor was amazing. She was not from my practice, so I didn't know what she would allow us to do, but she encouraged me to change positions and called the nurse midwife in. From there, my labor began to progress again. I no longer felt vulnerable, but felt empowered! I was in all-fours position and really starting to be able to work with the contractions and push effectively. I was eyeing getting out of bed, and our midwife encouraged me to do so. I got out of bed and continued to use my Womb Breathing. I felt like I was having the first dance with my baby. Womb Breathing helped me feel connected to her and my body. I embraced the contractions and squatted. Thirty minutes later, Lucy was born.

However, she did aspirate and was monitored in NICU for a few hours. Those hours apart were brutal, but still the practices of Calm Birth helped. We used the practice of Giving and Receiving, and I felt it helped us stay connected to our baby through those few hours we were apart.

Calm Birth truly helped us to feel confident in our birth process and to be connected as a family. I will always be grateful for this practice. We were able to have a peaceful birth, despite Lucy's difficulty breathing. I feel that this peaceful way of coming into the world helped her to overcome this challenge. I will always view our birth as our first dance together. I am so grateful that I do not have thoughts of pain, frustration, or fatigue when I think of our birth. It was natural, peaceful, and what we as a family needed and wanted it to be. I embraced the birth. It was an awesome ride.

Gahl Moriel

Baby: Gahl Moriel
Parents: Ellen and Douglas
Birth date: 8/7/03
Birth weight: 8 lb.15 oz.

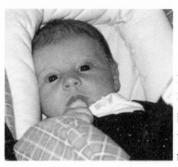

Photo by Ellen Moriel

Ellen had two sons, and she became pregnant again at the age of forty-two. Her husband, Douglas, is a respected doctor. From early in the pregnancy, Ellen fully applied the Calm Birth meditation, wanting a natural childbirth. The pregnancy proceeded beyond the due date, and Ellen continued the Calm Birth practices, sensing a special opportunity for communion with the child. Three weeks beyond the due date, she was able to continue Womb Breathing throughout labor. Afterward she said, "Deep breathing was natural and helped the birth process flow forward." She gave birth to a baby girl. Immediately after the delivery, the wide-eyed child made eye contact with Ellen, and then rested peacefully on her breast.

CB (Robert Bruce Newman, interviewer): The first thing that you mentioned that you wanted was calm, compared to what you experienced in your first two births. When were you introduced to Calm Birth?

Ellen: About four months ago, I received the CD.

CB: Concerning the Practice of Opening, how often have you been doing that?

Ellen: I've been pretty consistent. It's been about three or four times a week. I've been practicing the whole CD, all three practices. I've mostly been using the CD to practice, because that way I can focus the best. The texts [of the methods] are really interesting.

CB: In terms of where the language of the method brings you, what it facilitates for you, are you experiencing greater union in bonding with the child than in your previous births?

Ellen: I don't think so. It's been more my relationship with myself that's been changed—the understanding of my own empowerment—how to be more available to myself. Now I can understand what I'm thinking; I can notice what I'm thinking and where that's leading me. And then I come back to the practice and have thoughts that are more conducive to a calm birth.

CB: Does that have something to do with what you called "empowerment" in this practice?

Ellen: Absolutely. It's been very helpful. It gives me something solid to come back to. Now my body has been trained to get into that relaxation space. I think the baby definitely responds to that, understands that, knows that. In that way, the relationship has been deepened. I've always been very close with my babies.

CB: How often have you been doing the practice of Womb Breathing, as far as listening to the audioguide?

Ellen: The same as the Practice of Opening, at least three or four times a week. And then whenever I'm sitting down I remember; my body remembers the practice and does it.

CB: Besides the formal practice, how often do you do Womb Breathing?

Ellen: At least several times a day, I'll sit down to read a book to my kids, and as soon as I sit I remember to do the practice.... I think Womb Breathing is definitely amazing. It's a miracle what exactly can transpire. I take breathing for granted; but to really focus on it, to be under the practice, under the influence of the practice, what can happen is not an ordinary thing. I think any time I step out of my ordinary unconscious state it's a miracle. And to actually slow down and do the practice and experience it is calling in another energy. It kind of takes me to another level of waking up.

Therefore I appreciate my life, and life itself; I feel more alive. I'm more connected with the baby, more connected with everyone and everything.

CB: Would you say that Womb Breathing builds on your experience of Practice of Opening in giving you greater knowledge of your body and a more empowered sense of your own capability?

Ellen: Yes. I feel that Opening is the framework, the groundwork, and the two practices, Womb Breathing and Giving and Receiving, are a way to create it as a living thing, as something that's more accessible.... Giving and Receiving is interesting. I take some prenatal yoga classes. And I find myself thinking about the Giving and Receiving practice in those classes, when I'm with other pregnant women in the class, or when we run into each other in town. Some of them have issues.

CB: You mean conditions they have to deal with?

Ellen: Yes. And to be able to send them this—to give to them, to take in something and turn it into light—I think that's really good.

CB: Giving and Receiving is a famous healing practice from ancient wisdom. There've been amazing success stories with the practice. For the use of it in childbirth, does it add to the sense of empowerment you have in the other practices?

Ellen: I think that practice is really connected with people, feeling good intention, praying for them to resolve whatever their obstacles are.

Ethan

Baby: Ethan
Parents: Jeanne and Matthew
Birth date: 7/14/07
Birth weight: 7 lb. 2 oz.

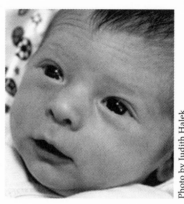

Photo by Judith Halek

Matthew and Jeanne found out that Jeanne was pregnant in November 2006. She was very focused on having a natural childbirth, without an epidural. She researched alternative breathing techniques for labor. When Jeanne was five months pregnant she found Judith Halek, a Calm Birth teacher. Jeanne and Matthew took a class from Judith to help prepare them for Ethan's birth. They got the Calm Birth CD from Judith. Jeanne listened to the CD almost every evening before falling asleep. She was able to attend a group practice with the Calm Birth CD, and to be part of a photo shoot for a magazine article on Calm Birth. Jeanne enjoyed doing Womb Breathing and said that she "loved the idea and practice of breathing vital life into her child."

Jeanne: When the moment arrived and labor started, I lay on the bed and breathed into my womb, as I learned from the Calm Birth CD. At first we played the Practice of Opening section of the CD; it helped me focus on each body part, which was a nice distraction from the discomfort of the contractions. I then moved to the Womb Breathing practice and found that I could breathe into my womb and then release the breath with a moaning sound. This, coupled with Matt pushing on my back and pulling on my hips, like Judith had taught us, really helped.

Ethan's birth was the most amazing experience. I feel so blessed to have had such a wonderful birth. Matt and I are really lucky to have found Judith and Eden, our doula, both of them Calm Birth teachers. Having Eden with us through labor and delivery made all the difference in keeping my birth calm. Between all the support, the great hospital staff, and Calm Birth, I feel that I was as ready as I could ever be to bring Ethan, my first child, into this world. I am so thankful for the wonderful birth, and I give thanks every day for such a fantastic child!

Cooper William

Baby: Cooper William
Parents: Chris and Molly
Birth date: 3/23/02
Birth weight: 8 lb. 9 oz.

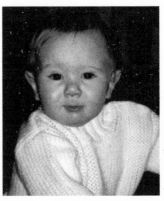

Photo by Chris Jorgensen

Molly had a physical problem that made intensive medical care necessary during her first childbirth. That resulted in having the birth pushed with pitocin, which then resulted in an epidural block. Molly felt this had been unnecessary, and she regretted not having the birth experience she had hoped for. There was no physical pain, but there were lingering unresolved feelings. For her second pregnancy, four years later, she was determined to eliminate medical interventions as much as possible. She had learned meditation as a child, and when her mother recommended the Calm Birth methods early in the pregnancy, Molly eagerly applied them and was able to experience an empowered birth.

CB (Whitney Wolf, interviewer): What is your memory of the first time you were introduced to the Calm Birth meditation?

Molly: My mother introduced me. She sent me the audioguide and an article about Calm Birth. I remember listening to the audio and thinking that some of it was things I already knew how to do like relaxing from your toes all the way up to your head. And just thinking that it was a really interesting thing to try.

CB: How far along in your pregnancy were you when you began using Calm Birth?

Molly: Maybe two months.

CB: What kind of previous meditation training have you done?

Molly: I had been taught how to meditate as a small child and would sort of practice it on and off as an adult. I'd learned different kinds of relaxation techniques.

CB: What was it you were looking for and wanted to find when you were introduced to the Calm Birth method?

Molly: I was just looking for anything that might help the labor process, tools to use that let me feel like I had something to be proactive with, in having a better attitude about the birth, more knowledge to feel more confident.

CB: Did you experience it that way?

Molly: Yes, I did. I felt like I had more of an understanding of and an appreciation of the labor process instead of it being just something hard that you go through. It's a simple part of the process that brings the baby to you. And then I felt that I was more confident because I had some extra tools.

CB: How would you describe the tools you learned from Calm Birth?

Molly: The ability to focus and the breathing were really helpful. The visualizing was very helpful, and some of the words I remembered from the audiocassette. Like the fact that the contractions are bringing the baby to you, so it is helpful to work with them, not against them. Also relaxing your whole body while in the middle of the pain.

CB: How often do you recall doing Practice of Opening before you gave birth?

Molly: It was sporadic, not really a regular thing. Sometimes it would be a couple of times per week, sometimes more.

CB: Usually in the evening?

Molly: Yes, usually in the evening right before going to bed.

CB: And how about the practice of Womb Breathing?

Molly: It was about the same. I'd alternate the methods. Sometimes I'd do the breathing for relaxation on my own without the CD. During pregnancy I woke up a lot during the night to go to the bathroom or because I was uncomfortable or something. I'd have a hard time going back to sleep, so I'd do the practice on my own to relax.

CB: Were you able to recall the meditation during the time that you were at the hospital?

Molly: Yes. I brought the CD and the audio player with me to the hospital, and during the first few hours I wore the headphones, playing the CD until things became more intense. Then I would sit in the rocking chair doing the breathing on my own.

CB: Was Womb Breathing helpful for your ability to recognize the difference between pain and suffering in labor?

Molly: Toward the end I didn't, because I was having a really hard time, right before I decided to have an epidural. I was having heavy contractions and yelling a lot. But I thought to myself that Womb Breathing was a way of going with it, so I was doing that to open up to the process. And then the contractions would be over and I would cry. It was really interesting to me. Yes, this is painful and I am going to express that. With my daughter's birth, I was given pitocin and an epidural, which was okay, and I just hung out till it was time to push and everything was kind of mellow and easy. But this time it was different. This time I really wanted to experience the true sense of labor, to see what that feels like.

CB: It sounds as though you were actively participating rather than watching it from afar.

Molly: Yes, exactly. And that's what I wanted. I wanted to try all of the things that you read about, standing, sitting, rocking in a chair, my husband right there with me so that we were there doing it together.

CB: As a result of your commitment to using Calm Birth, what stands out to you as being different between the first and second childbirth experiences?

Molly: With my first child, I guess I was not with the experience, and with my second child I was. The Calm Birth practice helped me with my anxiety levels and the ability to relax. It also helped me with some of the sleep problems that I had. And as I said, I felt more in control of the labor process. I had more information and more resources. That was the biggest thing, I think.

CB: Would you say that Calm Birth meditation helped you to experience a calmer childbirth?

Molly: Yes. Yes. I mean, you know that the labor process is an intense, painful thing, and I don't think that you can really get away from that. But while I was in the middle of it, I was feeling like this was what I really wanted to do, experience childbirth. Childbirth was a positive experience because I had information from the Calm Birth CD that was helpful, and I felt more confident in what I was doing and in how I was doing it. I was more in control.

CB: How did you feel more confident? What do you think was giving you the confidence?

Molly: I guess because I'd practiced the Calm Birth CD, I knew that I could get myself relaxed. I knew that I could do the Womb Breathing, and that would help me. And it did! It doesn't take the pain away, of course, but I just felt like I was a little more able to handle it. It wasn't as scary. It wasn't as unmanageable.

CB: Do you see benefits of Calm Birth in Cooper?

Molly: I think that he's calm in one sense in that he doesn't cry a lot and it is fairly easy to figure out what he needs … He hardly cries. He sleeps really well at night and he likes to giggle and move around.

CB: So as far as what was happening and what you were doing, were you aware of any synchronizing of the movements between you and Cooper during the contractions and delivery? Was there any kind of dialogue that you were aware of?

Molly: I remember the nurse was telling me that they showed me on the monitor where he was moving down. Then I thought, "Okay, along with my visualization of the contractions moving him down, I'm also going to open up, let him come out." It wasn't obvious that I was talking with him or doing visualization with him, but I was trying to have this flow going between us, and that is how I visualized it, that he was like a river.

CB: When the contractions were coming and caused your body to get tight, were you able to return to Womb Breathing?

Molly: Yes. I would notice the contraction would come and I could see the baby on the monitor coming and I could feel him, and when I would start to tense up, then I'd start breathing, breathing really deeply, and I'd close my eyes sometimes, or sometimes I'd look and focus on something else, or get my husband. I'd make a point of opening up and releasing him instead of tightening up more.

CB: Was Womb Breathing helpful for you to go on with those hours of labor?

Molly: Yes. Womb Breathing was a big part. I noticed that since I learned how to breathe more deeply, I instantly felt better.

CB: Please speak about breathing vital energy in the air. How was that helpful while you were doing Womb Breathing?

Molly: That was helpful in the sense that it was a visualization for me. As I was breathing, I visualized light coming into me and going down to him [Cooper, the baby].

CB: Did the visualization help you during contractions?

Molly: Well, it helped me by counteracting the pain. With pain there is a tendency of saying, "Pain is bad. This is bad because it hurts." This translates into something negative. Then doing Womb Breathing helped me to say, "I am bringing in what he and I both need, and continuing this movement to open up and to relax. This is part of what we need for him to come out."

CB: The first few hours of labor, were you able to return to Womb Breathing?

Molly: Yes. Maybe the first six or so hours and then the last hour I wasn't really able to do that. I got so tired. But I think the breathing meditation helped me stay in touch with my body and to listen to it, moving with the process rather than fighting it. It also helped to reduce anxiety and hold a focus.

CB: During pregnancy was there any kind of movement rhythm that you experienced with the baby?

Molly: Yes, the rhythm in movement with the Calm Birth breathing helped me to relax and synchronize with the baby before birth.

CB: Was Womb Breathing supportive of the natural movement for you during childbirth?

Molly: Yes. With Womb Breathing, if you're breathing deeply you can't be tensed up in your body. If you're really doing Womb Breathing, it helps you to relax, helping everything open and release.

CB: Did the Calm Birth methods give you a sense of self-empowerment during childbirth in the hospital?

Molly: Yes. I felt like I had more tools to use and something to actually practice so I could be more proactive and leading the process of childbirth instead of being led by the process. I felt more confident, like I could handle it and I knew what to do.

CB: What benefits, if any, do you see in your child from using the Calm Birth childbirth during pregnancy and throughout contractions and delivery?

Molly: I didn't notice so much with him during my pregnancy. I noticed more with me. I was able to be more relaxed, less anxious, and sleep better. I also believe that Calm Birth helped the process move forward more easily.

CB: What benefits, if any, do you see in yourself from using the Calm Birth practices?

Molly: I feel healthy and empowered.

CB: How do you feel healthy?

Molly: The Womb Breathing helps me relax, because I tend to have anxiety problems and stress. The breathing meditation does a lot to keep this sort of thing in check and I feel better, less stressed, with more energy, able to handle stress better.

CB: Can you sense that your prenatal Calm Birth efforts have given you and your child benefits that are long term?

Molly: I know that for me there will be long-term benefits, and I can assume that for Cooper there will be too. We will see how he develops. I feel I have the Calm Birth meditation forever.

CB: When you hold and feed Cooper, do you ever notice your body returning to the calming method?

Molly: Yes. I do the energy breathing.

CB: What do you notice in Cooper when you do that?

Molly: He will calm down. He used to sometimes get kind of irritated when I tried to feed him. Now he's making eye contact with me during nursing, which is very peaceful and nice.

Elias Grace

Baby: Elias Grace
Parents: Jennifer and Schiller
Birth date: 3/23/02
Birth weight: 7 lb. 9 oz.

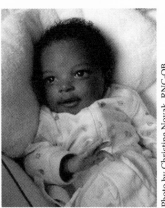

Photo by Christine Novak, RNC-OB

Jennifer: At twenty-two weeks pregnant I went to the doctor for an ultrasound, excited about the possibility of finding out whether I was having a boy or a girl. Instead, I discovered that I had almost no cervix left. Rather than being in the average range of 3–5 cm, my cervix was internally dilated and only 2 mm long. I knew this meant that the odds of carrying my baby to term were not in my favor.

I was immediately admitted to the hospital, and I spent the next twelve weeks on strict bed rest. During my first night at the hospital, I was introduced to Calm Birth by Christine Novak of the Calm Birth program. I instantly connected to Womb Breathing and Giving and Receiving.

Practicing these meditations while I was on bed rest allowed me to bond with my baby, manage my anxiety, and helped my body stay strong enough to support my pregnancy. My husband and

I would often listen to the Practice of Opening together during his visits, which helped him connect with our baby and prepared him to play a supportive role later on during labor. I wouldn't have made it through the long hospital stay without Christine and Calm Birth.

After such a difficult pregnancy, I grew increasingly anxious as my due date approached. I continued to practice the meditations daily to help prepare my mind, body, and baby for birth. While I was in labor, I found that I no longer needed to listen to the CD as a guide, because I automatically practiced the breathing and visualization I learned from Calm Birth to center and steady myself during each contraction. This allowed me to progress through labor feeling empowered and connected to the process.

After eleven hours of active labor, I gave birth to an alert, beautiful, healthy baby girl. I know that Calm Birth played a significant role in my successful pregnancy. I will always be grateful for this amazing resource.

McKane Scott

Baby: McKane Scott (Mickey)
Parents: Tamara and David
Birth date: 10/10/98
Birth weight: 8 lb. 8 oz.

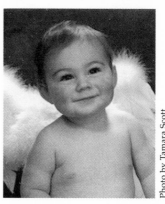

Photo by Tamara Scott

Tamara and David came to the Calm Birth program early in their first pregnancy. They applied the practices earnestly, desiring a natural childbirth. Unfortunately, an OB nurse at the hospital misjudged the position of the baby in the uterus, not understanding that it was breech, and encouraged premature pushing during labor. This resulted in various difficulties and ended in a cesarean birth. However, Tamara was able to maintain an exceptional calm and clarity, which benefited all concerned. As the following description relates, she considered it an empowered birth. The child emerged calm and aware.

Tamara: My water broke, and I realized I was going into labor. And it was my first time. I was thinking, "I'm going to have this period where the contractions are going to be really slow and calm and I'm going to play the Calm Birth CD, and listen to it." As soon as my water broke, I was pacing the house. Altered. My contractions were really intense. I was told afterwards it was just because of the breech position. He was against my pelvis. So I labored for eighteen hours. No drugs. Thank God I had Dave and my other two birth coaches breathing in my face telling me not to push. That was another thing: because of the position, I wanted to push for a lot longer than most people do. And then I ended up having a C-section.

CB (Whitney Wolf, interviewer): Did they attempt to turn the baby at all?

David: I think they didn't diagnose his position until much later.

Tamara: I didn't have a chance to meditate. As I said, as soon as my water broke I was pacing and basically I walked up and down that hospital the whole eighteen hours. I couldn't sit. But I think the part that helped me was to stay in control. To know that I could breathe into the pain, not let the pain take over my body, freak me out, and feel out of control. And, now that I think about it, the Calm Birth meditation was very helpful. A lot of women, if it's their first time, won't know what they're going to experience. Nothing prepares you. You get fight or flight and you're thinking, "Okay, here we go." I don't know. Dave, you think I remained pretty calm? Despite the positioning?

David: Yeah, I think you were great. It was extremely valuable information and entirely positive in all respects. We were 100 percent committed to the Calm Birth practice.

Tamara: Yes.

David: You incorporated it partly into how you went through the birth. We weren't talking about Calm Birth while we were going through it, but it was in our psyche somewhere.

Tamara: In our systems.

CB: What was your first impression of the Calm Birth class, do you remember?

Tamara: Yeah. I felt empowered. I thought, "This is great, this information." That was the first class we ever took.

CB: Did you attend with her, David?

David: Yes.

Tamara: So I think that was my main feeling of control: that I don't have to give my power away to the doctor, which I think I normally would have. If I didn't have the Calm Birth training, I would have been so freaked out, like, "This is my first time," and I would have given them more power than was necessary. So that part really helped me. That was my first impression of the class, about empowerment. Karen, my doctor, afterwards came up to me and said, "You know, I just want to say how impressed I am with how awake and aware you were." It made her feel comfortable. She knew that I wanted a vaginal delivery. I think she felt bad that didn't happen.

David: Tamara's personality and the way she does things is not calm, not meditative. She usually steps up to a challenge more in an intense manner. Which I mean, you can do, I think, at that level of meditation. As I said, I think you can be in a meditative state to a certain extent while you're going through this far more physical activity.

Tamara: Exactly, and I feel like I was. I didn't feel so out of it. I was directing these guys to breathe with me.

David: There was no screaming or hysterics. Everything was very calm the whole time, but she had to stay active, on the move.

Tamara: Yes, I just couldn't sit. I kept in a movement thing.

CB: I'd say you were very successful, Mom.

Tamara: I think I was. I have a beautiful, healthy boy. I like to think it's all perfect, with what was supposed to happen. It was an incredible thing.

CB: Do you feel that Calm Birth may have been helpful in dealing with pain and fear issues?

Tamara: Yes, it did really resonate with me in thinking about the fear of labor. I was afraid of that. But I do know that Calm Birth, just by listening to the CD, you know: don't be afraid of the pain. You know, breathe with the contraction. Don't go against the contraction. That part of it made a lot of sense to me. Every time I would feel a contraction come on, I was prepared for it. I was not totally welcoming the contraction, but I was leaning into it, and breathing into it, which I think helped me feel not totally out of control, screaming. So that part was very helpful.

CB [to David]: What did you experience when you did the practices with Tamara? What do you remember?

David: I remember doing it with the intention to provide the right environment, or create the right intention for the delivery of our baby. I'd say I experienced putting forth the right intentions with it.

Tamara: And that's how it was in the labor room too. Dave was really present, breathing with me. And it was great. For the whole labor thing, I hope that the next time around I'll have a vaginal delivery and experience that feeling, but I'm okay if that doesn't happen too. It doesn't have to be a particular plan. I was proud of myself. And lying on the birthing table I was smiling. The doctor said, "Look, you're smiling." I felt radiant even then ... That's my experience. I was awake and talking. I felt connected to the doctors. It was a great experience.

CB: So as you reflect back on this, do you feel kind of like there was something about the spiritual aspect for you in the Calm Birth methods?

Tamara: Let me think. I know with the Calm Birth CD, when I would listen, it did take me into a space I loved, the tuning into my womb and trying to visualize the light, and that little being growing inside of me. It was just incredible. The whole time, I was thinking I was having a girl. So I wasn't totally aware [laughs], because it was a boy. And then of course we felt that when we conceived Mickey, that it was a conscious conception. We were totally aware of what we were doing, of our intention. I did visualize a spirit kind of hovering above us, choosing us as its parents in this lifetime. Things like that would come to my mind. During the laboring process, I remember at one point not resisting, but feeling, fear; then I realized I was feeling that in my body, and I said that I want to release that. I said, "I'm afraid to be a mother. I've never been a mother before." The responsibility was huge, and I was aware of that during the contractions. I looked at the nurse, and I said something, and I saw tears in her eyes. I said, "Okay, I'm surrendering now. I'm ready to be a mom." Even when we're talking about it, it gives me chills because it was such a conscious place.

CB: After taking the weekend intensive Calm Birth class, how often did you do the practices at home?

Tamara: I knew I couldn't commit to doing it every day, but it was always in my awareness. We did the practices together a few times a week. I think that the nurse who was first there with us at the hospital would have loved the Calm Birth practices. I think it's great for the nurses who are there, because the doctors don't show up until the end.

CB [to David]: Could you envision the baby actually forming in Tamara's belly?

David: From the first moment, when we decided to conceive, we had a clear vision of creating a baby, at the exact moment we started trying. So that part was never difficult to envision.

CB: So you had that spiritual experience at conception?

David: Conscious conception experience, yes.

Tamara: I don't know if it was at exactly the same time. Spiritually we were trying, envisioning the child at the same time. He's the ultimate joy, for sure. I never knew how much I could love.

CB: Did you or David have any meditation experience previous to the Calm Birth training?

Tamara: I had a very brief introduction to Buddhist meditation. Marina, one of the birth coaches, did a Buddhist practice at her home, and I participated in that a little. I worked at that for a couple of months, and then I got pregnant. I did enjoy it.

CB: Do you feel like the Calm Birth practice created any sort of direct bonding with the baby prior to birth, for you and with David?

Tamara: Yes, definitely yes. When I did the practice and I pictured the womb, and sending light to it, visualizing, it definitely was great, connecting me with what was going on inside my body, in a deeper level, feeding those blessings to it. That was really nice.

CB: How fortunate for the baby to have parents like you.

Tamara: Yes. To be present, that's what I wanted. I wanted to be as present as possible in his life. Because you often hear parents say, "It goes by like this" [snaps her fingers]. You blink your eyes and then they're in high school...

David: He's a very confident, comfortable baby.

Tamara: I think that's because of Calm Birth and just being that conscious when he was being conceived and during the whole pregnancy; that's why he is so comfortable... I did the energy meditation, which I visualized would help a baby in the womb. I did the Womb Breathing and sent the baby that energy. And I definitely was breathing that way as much as possible during the whole labor. I mean, I had to.... I want to say that Calm Birth really enforced for me that I didn't have to do drugs. Which was great to have that. I would have friends who would say that you're crazy to not use painkilling drugs, just do it, like it's no big deal. But I think if we have empowered mamas, we have empowered babies [laughs].

Elias John

Baby: Elias John
Parents: Jennifer and Max
Birth date: 2/25/99
Birth weight: 8 lb. 4 oz.

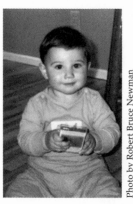

Photo by Robert Bruce Newman

Jennifer and Max wanted to bring meditation into their lives. It was Jennifer's pregnancy and their desire for a natural childbirth that brought them to meditation in the Calm Birth program. They succeeded, meditating with their child in the womb throughout the pregnancy, labor, and delivery. Then they knew that meditation would be a good postnatal family path.

CB (Robert Bruce Newman, interviewer): You really applied the Calm Birth practice not only in the weekend training program but also on through the weekly follow-up classes. We know you were putting it in your systems. With respect to the reclining practice, we've had couples do that with the man visualizing the baby in himself. Did you do that, Max?

Max: Yes. It was pretty amazing. We used good thoughts and listened to the technique. Jennifer was doing it every night, but I was doing it probably every other night, right before bed usually.

CB: Did you have that experience of imagining the womb inside yourself?

Max: Yes. It was pretty awesome, amazing… It allowed me to get a close bond with my child, and it was nice that I could actually experience the pregnancy for all of us.

CB: How often did you practice Womb Breathing, Jennifer?

Jennifer: I did the practices every night: meditating and focusing on my womb, focusing on the child. I developed a much stronger bond. It felt like I was feeding him energy and he was responding to it. So it felt like even though he was still in the womb, I was caring for him. Our relationship was already being established. So, like when he came out, it was like, "I know you."

CB: You said you were sending him energy. You were one with him. Did you feel that you were in meditation with the baby?

Jennifer: Yes.

Max: Oh yes. We listened to the CD, and that was our meditation practice for us. Instead of meditating on yourself, to focus your breath and all that, it was more focused on him, less on myself.

Jennifer: I didn't use the meditation techniques during the whole labor. I did use them more with the relaxing of the body. I did the practice of breathing directly into the area of the pain then, and it helped.

CB: Did you find that Calm Birth was a complement to what you were doing in your hospital class?

Jennifer: Definitely. I was going to try everything to have a natural childbirth. I wanted to really experience it.

CB: How often did you do the Womb Breathing practice?

Jennifer: I think about three times a week. It was early in the pregnancy that we started the Calm Birth program, in the fall. I was barely showing ... By the time of the birth, the breathing practice was like an unconscious thing. It just became natural.

CB: So it had become like second nature?

Jennifer: Yes. And I think that definitely helped during the labor. I didn't even go to the hospital until I was 8 cm dilated. I mean, most people go in earlier than that.

CB: And your water broke at that point?

Jennifer: No, it never did.

Max: They thought of delivering him in it, but then at the last second the contractions started slowing down. They said it actually stopped in some cases. So they broke her water.

Jennifer: Yes, so I know the deep breathing helped throughout … Yes, it was great. I couldn't have asked for anything better.

Max: There was all this smiling and then the baby came out, and the doctor then came in just to catch the baby.

CB: Would you say that it was an easy birth?

Jennifer: Oh no. I definitely went through some serious pain.

CB: There were some hard contractions?

Jennifer: Oh yes. Then pushing was hard. It wasn't all just breathing. But then my contractions stopped in the pushing phase. That's when I think the primal stuff came out [laughs].

CB: What made you think that it was time to go to the hospital?

Jennifer: That's when I realized, "Gosh, I'm really in pain here." My contractions were building. They were not consistently five minutes apart. It was like ten minutes, then three minutes. Just not consistent. But it was fine. It definitely was liberating. We look back and say, "Wow, we did that all by ourselves." It was just a process I took my body through…. I've had friends who barely knew they were in labor. It wasn't that easy. But the only time I felt fear maybe was when I heard they wouldn't let you push for more than two hours and it was maybe getting to that time. The contractions weren't coming. So that was the only time I felt like,

"Uh-oh, I hope the hospital doesn't want me to do a C-section." But I never really had the sense of what I'd call fear. When you give in to fear, the problems start to arise.

CB: I think that's the most important thing, for a child to be born without fear. It doesn't mean to be born without pain. It sounds like you worked with the pain well.

Jennifer: Yes. I could accept it.

CB: That affects the child importantly.

Jennifer: The doctor said he was very alert.

Max: The minute he was out of the womb, he was wide-eyed, looking around. I didn't expect that. I think that's due to the calmness of the labor.

[Baby gleeful. Everyone laughs.]

CB: So you were instructed that meditation wasn't just for pre-birth and birth. The more you continue to meditate, the more it will help the child in every way.

Jennifer: Max and I were thinking: you do all the prep work for the birth experience and then the hard part comes afterwards. I think meditation's really good for him, because he needs to calm down.

Emily Rose

Baby: Emily Rose
Parents: Marie and Lee
Birth date: 5/2/99
Birth weight: 4 lb. 4 oz.

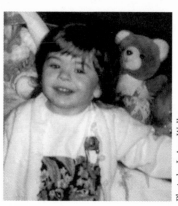

Photo by JoAnn Walker

Marie was a thirty-seven-year-old woman with many medical problems when she became pregnant. She had prayed for a child in spite of the fact that she was told it would be impossible for her to conceive after she had been treated surgically for ovarian cancer. She was told that if she did conceive, it was unlikely that the child would be born, and if it was, she was warned, it might have serious health problems. When she did become pregnant, she was encouraged to terminate the pregnancy. She refused. She was referred to the Calm Birth program both because Marie expressed interest in meditation and because her OB doctor thought that the Calm Birth program might help her in her high-risk pregnancy. Marie often did the Calm Birth practices for several hours a day.

She and her husband Lee were exemplary in their commitment. They succeeded in having a natural childbirth. Marie became a teacher in the Calm Birth program and helped bring the method to many women the program may not have reached.

CB (JoAnn Walker, RN, interviewer): Would you please tell us your medical history before your pregnancy?

Marie: Okay. Because I was born with hydrocephalus, I have had several shunt revisions [a brain surgery that inserts a plastic tube into the brain and body cavities to drain the excess cranial fluid], and I have intractable migraine syndrome, which means I don't know what it's like not to have a headache. Thanks to a lot of different things, I can make my migraines much better. I have diabetes, chronic fatigue, TMJ, and a sleep disorder, narcolepsy, where I either sleep all the time or don't sleep at all, for weeks and weeks at a time. I have brain damage because of all the shunt revisions.

CB: When did the hydrocephalus start?

Marie: From birth. I had my first operation when I was twenty-seven days old. I'm not quite sure how many skull operations I've had, but I know it's over thirty.

CB: When were you diagnosed with diabetes?

Marie: 1984.

CB: And your husband had been gone for a while? Almost three years?

Marie: Almost three.

CB: But you were still married, and he came home. There was supposedly no chance of you getting pregnant, right?

Marie: Virtually no chance, right.

CB: Yet it happened.

Marie: Yes. That's a real miracle.

CB: So here you are, you're thirty-seven years old and you've been told you can't get pregnant. You have multiple medical problems. You're on a variety of different medicines. And you're seven months pregnant?

Marie: Right at twenty-seven weeks. The doctor asked that I get tested right away, with ultrasound and stuff, because of all the medication I'm on, and all the different conditions. He wanted to know if abortion was an option. I told him it's just not an option with me.

I have only one fallopian tube and one ovary because of ovarian cancer. So it's a miracle that I'm pregnant.

CB: Other than the surgeries for your shunts, you've had major abdominal surgery?

Marie: Yes.

CB: So you choose to work with an OB/GYN, and to continue your pregnancy.

Marie: Absolutely. It's a miracle. Because of all my medical conditions, and because of my history, I'm working very closely with my personal physician, and two different doctors in OB/GYN.

CB: Marie, you're considered a high-risk pregnancy. Why will you probably need a medical center for the birth?

Marie: Because the hydrocephalus could go haywire.

CB: Do you have more fluid because you're pregnant?

Marie: Yes. They don't have a whole lot of knowledge yet. I was one of the first ones to ever get a shunt. What they do know is that pregnancies tend to clog shunts. But it also may be fine. I'm just going to keep doing the meditation.

CB: Marie, you and your husband, Lee, attended the six-hour Calm Birth training and then attended the weekly hour support groups. How often do you do the Calm Birth practices?

Marie: Well, I use the Calm Birth CD. I use the Practice of Opening to help me relax. Sometimes if the migraines aren't too bad, I practice the whole CD. Sometimes I spend hours in the bathtub listening to the CD over and over again.

CB: So the Calm Birth CD is helping you with relaxation. Does it help with your headaches?

Marie: Depending on the magnitude of the headache.

CB: In terms of doing the Calm Birth practices, have you noticed any changes with the baby? Have you noticed her respond?

Marie: Oh yes. She relaxes and settles down most of the time when I practice.

CB: You're teaching the Calm Birth method to some of your friends. How is that going?

Marie: We really like it because there is the CD. There is comfort in repetition. It's like listening to your favorite music. You can relax, and it calms you sooner than just trying to calm yourself.

Lee: Marie's a very special woman. It's a miracle that she got pregnant, with these different kinds of medications she's on. Medications and hormone shots will prevent a woman from getting pregnant. And in this particular case, God must want this baby to happen. Doctors told her they were giving us less than 5 percent of a chance for us to have a child. But with the Calm Birth meditation, it's helped us get closer together. And it helps us get closer to our child. That, we can relate with. The baby will teach us a lot of things when she gets here. She's going to teach us how to be parents. And we're going to teach her to have fun in life and to help other people when she gets older. The Calm Birth practices are helping us with our emotional needs. The practice helps us relax our physical bodies, and also helps us with our emotions, when we go through excitement. Tension, fear, and frustration rise up sometimes. The Calm Birth practices help us deal with it and realize that this life is a miracle that we're going through.

Postnatal Interview

Baby: Emily Rose (approximately five weeks
premature at 33½ weeks)
Parents: Marie and Lee
Birth date: 5/2/99
Birth weight: 4 lb. 4 oz.

CB (Robert Bruce Newman, interviewer): Marie, were the Calm Birth methods an assistance to you in stopping your premature labor?

Marie: Yes. Yes. Primarily because I knew from practicing the Calm Birth CD and the classes how to relax my body. That's very important.

CB: You were in labor but didn't realize it; can you tell us about this?

Marie: Yes. It didn't start being strong until about midnight. And then she was born at 6:25 in the morning, so it was a short and easy labor.

CB: Did Womb Breathing really help?

Marie: Yes. It was with me throughout. There were times when the pains would get bad enough so that I'd forget the Womb Breathing, and they had me pant like a puppy, and I found that all that did was make me feel like I was hyperventilating. So I remembered the teaching from the Calm Birth CD, and that helped me through labor immensely…. The practice had become like second nature.

CB: So you were in the hospital, in labor, and the breathing meditation, you say, was active in you spontaneously?

Marie: That is correct.

CB: What about the pushing part?

Marie: The more I was able to push, the less painful the contractions were, and I was able to push her out relatively quickly, because I had fresh air and I had normal breathing.

CB: What about the fears you had because of all the things that could go wrong?

Marie: I had been experiencing panic attacks the last couple of days, since I had been home from [the first premature labor visit to] the hospital, and I practiced the calm breathing then, and it helped a lot.

Gabriel and Emily

Babies: Gabriel Frederick
and Emily Natalia
Parents: Maria and Joseph
Birth date: 11/14/11
Birth weights: 6 lb. 7 oz.
and 6 lb. even

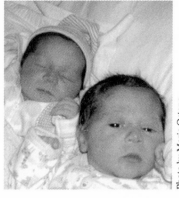

Photo by Maria Octano

Maria: No one thought I would go full term, but I did! They [the hospital staff] scared me into thinking that the twins were going to come really early, and I got a lot of pressure to induce. I finally had to say yes to them doing a stripping of the membranes, and when I got to the hospital they broke my water. I gave birth in under three hours. It was a fight, since I didn't appreciate the treatment I got. They rushed me, and I literally had to close my legs when I got to the hospital since I wanted to labor a bit and let the water bag break on its own.

The Calm Birth practice, along with Marci, my doula, helped me stay relaxed and focused. I didn't get to listen to my CD until the last month of the pregnancy, but during that month I did do it about three times a day to keep from getting anxious. Her voice [on the audioguide] was really soothing, and even though the delivery and labor were rushed and chaotic, I was able to maintain some sort of equilibrium inside myself.

Nicholas

Baby: Nicholas
Parents: Nora and Javier
Birth date: 5/26/99
Birth weight: 8 lb. 7 oz.

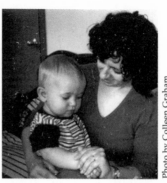

Photo by Colleen Graham

Nora's first child was born in Argentina. She was anxious and isolated throughout that pregnancy, with no support and no childbirth education. Her husband wasn't allowed to be with her at the birth, and she didn't know any of the birthing personnel at the hospital. She was given anesthesia and woke up the day after the child had been delivered by C-section. Several years later, with three months remaining in her second pregnancy, she met two of the Calm Birth teachers and began practicing the method. Her second birth experience was very different from her first. As she tells us, she was able to have the birth she always wanted.

CB (Robert Bruce Newman, interviewer): What inspired you to come to the Calm Birth program?

Nora: I was trying to have a better pregnancy than with my first child. I was trying to have a happier pregnancy. The first time, in Argentina, I was very nervous and insecure. The last month was sort of a nightmare. My mother wasn't with me, and I missed her. I felt anxious. There were many nights I couldn't sleep, not just sleepless, but sad, and thinking and thinking and thinking. Then I had a C-section. I'd never seen the doctor before. It was a very bad experience.

CB: I remember you saying you didn't have much of a birth experience. They gave you anesthetic and you woke up much later.

Nora: Yes. My husband wasn't allowed to be with me. I had no support at all.

CB: So this time you wanted to have much more support, and to be more empowered.

Nora: Yes. I had met with Colleen* and Sandra† on my birthday, and they said that I didn't have to do the same thing twice [C-section]. Then everything changed. I started relaxing and enjoying the pregnancy. I began to study at the university, to take more classes.

CB: The title, "Calm Birth," did that mean something to you?

Nora: Yes. But you have to be ready. Colleen said to sit down and relax, and I did. I wasn't a perfect student, like doing it every morning, but I did the practice.

CB: How often?

Nora: I had had a virus and was sick for two weeks, but when Colleen asked me to sit down and do the practice, from the first time I did it I felt better. It allowed me to not think, to put my mind at ease. To relax. I began to sleep better. I did it several times a week.

CB: In the reclining meditation practice, you go right into the womb with the child.

Nora: Yes.

CB: Did that help you in terms of actually making contact with the child?

Nora: Yes. Definitely. He is more outgoing than my first child. We had conversations when he was in the womb. He moved a lot. We felt very close. I remember the practices. The one where you lie down

*Colleen Graham is a doula, educator, and Calm Birth teacher who served as Nora's doula.
†Sandra Bardsley, RN, FACCE, LCCE, CD, is a midwife, educator, and Calm Birth board member.

allowed me to relax and have good sleep at night, which I couldn't do with my first pregnancy. This time I was able to just focus on the baby and myself and the pregnancy.

CB: You mentioned about actually communicating with him in the womb, like speaking with him directly, in telepathic communication with the child.

Nora: Yes. I'll remember the joy of the communication. My first birth was so heavy. I'll never forget how joyful this second childbirth has been.

CB: Did the language on the Calm Birth CD enable you to reach Nicholas and meditate with him?

Nora: Yes. Probably that's true. We're very connected. I think that the last two weeks, when the first contractions came, I put on the CD and it really, really helped me. It relaxed me and helped me to focus on what was going on.

CB: Can you tell us about the birth?

Nora: The labor was long. It ended up being a cesarean, even though I wanted a natural birth. The breathing practices from the CD were implemented during this time. I was in labor for two days. Finally I decided to have the C-section because the labor just wasn't working out. Because I felt relaxed, I felt okay with that, and he is a gifted child. That is communication, isn't that it? He just loves communicating. It doesn't matter what age they are, he just loves to be with people and he expresses his feelings perfectly well. His smile is something beautiful.

CB: So maybe the best thing for him was that communication that you gave him before birth. It was like a prayer being answered to bring him to his greater potential.

Nora: He is very responsive to music. And he's so beautiful. The doctor looked at him and said he was such a beautiful newborn. Exquisite and so nice and alert. His eyes were looking around. He wasn't cranky. Just an open baby.

CB: In the Calm Birth class at the hospital, we talked with you about the method of breathing energies in the air to benefit the child in the womb. Were you able to do that during labor?

Nora: Yes. The labor was hard. I really tried the deep breathing. When I wasn't doing that, I tried to focus, but I was busy with my first son the whole day. So I put the CD on and communicated with the child, saying that he was really wanted. I told him he had a mother, a father, and a brother here who really want him, and love him. I did that every day. When I felt a contraction, I was playing the CD and saying, "Oh, we're so right for you. It's okay to come out." I did the deep breathing method during the labor. I couldn't imagine not doing it.

CB: After you were given the CD at your birthday party, how long did it take you to realize that the meditation was useful?

Nora: Two tries. The first time, I thought it was okay, not so bad; but the second time, I was sick, and so worried about the baby. When you're sick and pregnant, the only thing you can take is Tylenol. But the audiocassette really helped me. It helped me to relax. That night, I could just think of the baby and myself, and it was okay. To me, after the first pregnancy, feeling relaxed was a big thing. With the first birth I couldn't sleep for nights and nights.

CB: When you went to sleep at night, did the energy of the breathing practice stay with you?

Nora: Yes, absolutely.

CB: Because of that relaxation, were you more confident about your pregnancy?

Nora: My pregnancy had a before and after. Before I met with Colleen and Sandra and got the CD, I was insecure and afraid. I thought my first childbirth experience was repeating. But with the Calm Birth practice, I realized I don't have to do that again. I relaxed and took the classes. I'd been so afraid that I didn't even mention to people that I was pregnant, because the first experience had been so bad.

CB: So it sounds like your birthday party with Colleen and Sandra was the turning point.

Nora: It was like a special club that women have in being a mother. We were together in the joy of having a baby. I'd been sick, and I went home and listened to the CD and everything was different. Amazing. And my husband was very involved.

Colleen (CB interviewer): I remember him saying, "Nora, remember your breathing. Breathe like you were guided on the CD. Do Womb Breathing."

Nora: I tried it in different positions. The best one for me was on my knees. I was 100 percent focused. And my husband was right there, with his memory of the CD. We did it all together. I couldn't imagine him not being there. He was the most committed, most dedicated husband I could imagine. And this is the product [holding up her baby, Nicholas].

CB: Nora, when do you think a pregnant woman should start practicing these methods?

Nora: I think the CD is really good, and I think women need to use it whenever they feel ready to have this commitment with themselves. As I learned during the famous conversation that day, being pregnant is a very special moment. It's okay to feel and to show everybody and to be proud of that. It is a very special moment. These nine months are a very special period in your lifetime. Because I was busy with my first child, the CD helped me focus on the pregnancy, on the child inside me. So I thought, "I want to be with the unborn child tonight, so I will put on the CD and practice and be with him." I'm sure his open style is related to that experience. He had a different mother than my first child. With Nicholas, the eye contact and the communications are easier.

CB: He's calmer.

Nora: Exactly. They say the CD helps you focus on your pregnancy, to stop everything, to say, "I am pregnant. This is happening to me now, and I will live this period of my life in the best way I can." The Calm Birth CD helps with that. I know pregnant women who act like nothing's happening.

Colleen: I noticed that when Nora would get kind of uptight, Javier, her husband, would say to her, "Play the CD and relax," and it would help. It gave him something good to do.

Nora: Yes.

CB: So your husband's involvement and support during this childbirth was very important.

Nora: Yes. The experience with the first child was awful for both of us. There, the doctors excluded him [Javier] from the birth.

CB: The intention while creating the Calm Birth CD was that it's for both the mother and the father.

Nora: Yes, the CD really helps the father get closer to the child.

CB: How was Colleen there for you during your second pregnancy?

Nora: Colleen was my doula during the process. She was with me throughout the pregnancy and then for the three days before the birth. She was at the hospital with Javier and myself, exactly reminding me of my breathing.... I told Colleen that I saw a movie that when a baby was born, they sang "Happy Birthday," and I loved that. And Colleen said we could do that. So we were in the recovery room, after the C-section, and everyone was happy, including the baby. And Colleen said, "Remember the birthday song!" And we all sang "Happy Birthday" for him. The nurses were there. It was wonderful. The welcoming was very bonding.

Makai

Baby: Makai
Parents: Mysty and John
Birth date: 6/10/99
Birth weight: 8 lb. 3 oz.

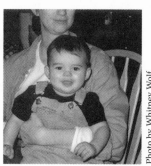

Photo by Whitney Wolf

Mysty and John were young honey farmers. It was their first pregnancy. They wanted a natural childbirth and connected with an OB doctor who was very supportive of the Calm Birth program. In preparing for the birth with the Calm Birth practice, Mysty and John had what they called fulfilling meditation experiences. They worked together closely as a birth team, using the meditation throughout labor and delivery. They were very happy with the birth.

Mysty: We were in our twenty-eighth week. We were looking for ways of giving birth where we could do it naturally. And I saw an announcement for a Calm Birth seminar. Up until that time, I guess I was insecure about giving birth. I wondered whether I could do it without interventions. That wasn't possible with some doctors, but it was very possible with other doctors. So we were trying to figure out a way to do it without interventions, and we came across the Calm Birth announcement and we decided to take the seminar. It was very enlightening. It was two days long, and we learned a lot. It was very insightful.

John: We learned and affirmed.

Mysty: Yes, learned and affirmed.

John: A lot of it was things we already believed. You gave back to us what we knew.

Mysty: I started using the CD, especially in the evening before I went to bed. And I actually had some really great meditation experiences. I never used to meditate much, so that was really cool.

CB (Robert Bruce Newman and Whitney Wolf, interviewers): You were supposed to visualize the womb within yourself. Did you do that?

John: Yes, we did that. We did that practice more than anything.

CB: You felt natural doing that?

John: Yes, absolutely. Definitely. I felt the connection with her.

CB: Did you notice any difference in your experience after beginning the Womb Breathing practice?

Mysty: The only changes were that I felt more confident. Before, I didn't know what to do. I was still frightened. With the meditation it was almost like I had tools. I was armed with something I could use. Before that, I had been at the mercy of whatever.

John: If it was only to make a person confident, that's a great thing to do for somebody. But I think it's more than that. Because if you really establish that connection with the unborn child, you focus your energy on that, being welcoming and nurturing.

CB: We know you had a quick labor. You had labor contractions, and you called Dr. Olsen and you went straight to the hospital?

Mysty: Dr. Olsen said it probably wouldn't be that day. It would probably be the next day or the next day. It could be that day, but it probably will be the next day. But we were primed for it because we knew.

John: Yes. I said, "I'm not starting any chore that I can't stop right away." I knew it was that close. I felt a special awareness. Some of it probably comes from the meditation and having a good bond before he was out. Also the high level of communication between the two of us.

CB: Mysty, did you say that the labor wasn't hard?

Mysty: It was relatively easy.

John: Not that easy.

Mysty: Yes, I catch myself saying it was easy, but I was in labor all day long. I was really excited.

John: The stuff that lasted all day long was mild. We went shopping.

Mysty: Dr. Olsen said go home. She was aware of where we live [twenty miles away from Ashland Community Hospital] and how long it would take to get back into the hospital. We went home. I called my mom. She said to walk around, but I was tired. We'd been home about half an hour. I decided to lie down and do some meditation.

John: She did some good visualization.

Mysty: Yes, I did some visualizations of my cervix opening. It was while I was doing that that my water broke, and I went into intense labor. We went back to the hospital by the back roads.

CB: Were there times when labor was happening that you remembered to do Womb Breathing?

Mysty: I didn't have to remember. I just did it, automatically. It's like I knew to do it. I'd catch myself doing the energy breathing already. And John was helping me as I kept breathing calm.

John: It did get a little difficult, because we wanted to incorporate Womb Breathing in the delivery, but at a certain point they said they wanted her to push at it and do the panting. That was weird for me.

Mysty: Yes, that was hard for you, the way the nurses pushed.

John: Everyone was looking at me like, "How come you're not coaching the pant breathing?" and I talked about this other kind of breathing we were trying to do.

Mysty: In the hard part of my labor, I was in the Jacuzzi. I would start to pant when they told me to pant, and then I would slow down and just try to focus into the calm breathing.

CB: They would say, "Pant, fast-breathe," and you would want to slow down and focus?

Mysty: Yes.

John: If the nurses on duty had listened to the CD, it would have been different. But Mysty kept doing the deep, calm breathing anyway, and we had a perfect natural birth. What I liked the most about the Calm Birth program is that before the baby is born, you can communicate, bless, and give it energy.

Ari and Ivory

Ari: Birth date: 7/28/06
Birth weight: 7 lb. even
Ivory: Birth date: 1/16/10
Birth weight: 6 lb. 6 oz.
Parents: Denise and Sam

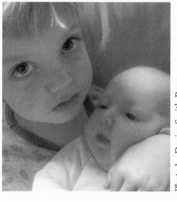

Photo by Denise Smith-Rowe

CB (Robert Bruce Newman, interviewer) [to make a wonderful love story short and sweet]: I taught vase breathing meditation to Sam, the son of my closest friend. Sam loved meditation and practiced it often. We met from time to time and talked about his practice. Then he met the love of his life, in Nicaragua, of all places. They grew up six miles apart in Oregon, went to the same high school, but weren't close, and then met and fell in love in a faraway place years later. Sam taught Denise vase breathing, which she was very interested in, and they practiced together. Then very quickly Denise became pregnant. It was like they breathed the baby in. They sent me an email and asked me about doing vase breathing during the pregnancy.

Sam: Robert sent us an email with a written version of Womb Breathing, and from the beginning Denise began breathing light and life into our little boy. During meditation I would do the same. It was such a wonderful feeling to be intending freedom and energy towards my unborn child. I knew God was sending us this child as a gift, wrapped in Denise, already in a perfect state. This was an amazing, calming sensation.

We returned to Hugo and spent the six months before Ari's birth working on the garden, fixing up our little studio building, and enjoying our time together. I have clear images of Denise upstairs listening to the Calm Birth CD, and I was feeling lucky to have a woman using her intention to support our coming child. Her pregnancy was a truly beautiful time.

A midwife came to our house to assist with the birth. Denise was so strong and positive. Her father had died about a year earlier of brain cancer, and we felt the baby as her father's energy being reborn, in a way. There were definitely some powerful woman yells during the birth, but I saw no fear or worry from Denise. She was amazing. Ari came so fast that I was able to catch him since the other midwife didn't have time to make the birth. Denise needed eighteen stitches due to the speed of Ari's delivery, but she was so happy she didn't even know that she tore. Her face of joy was so beautiful when she saw her baby boy. I held him quietly in my arms, looking into his eyes, his deep, unwavering stare, while the midwife stitched up Denise. I was blessed.

As Ari grew, his awareness and thoughtfulness were quickly apparent. He was speaking Spanish in Nicaragua before he was two. Ever observant, he loved to eat out of the garden and just be with us. When he was three, he told Denise, "You can meditate if you want to." We definitely saw Ari as our little teacher.

CB: When I was told what Ari had said to his mother about meditation, a stunning statement from a three-year-old, I decided to visit the little wise man to show him a photograph. It's a photo of a three-year-old Tibetan baby Buddha, a reincarnated master, sitting in meditation posture, smiling, with his young monk attendant sitting beside him. They really looked to me like they both knew how to meditate well. I asked Ari to look at the photograph closely. I said that the little boy was a baby Buddha. I asked Ari to look and tell me if he could see that the little boy knew how to meditate. Ari looked carefully, and we leaned toward him to hear what he might say. In the quietest clear voice I've ever heard, he said, "Yes."

Sam: When Ari was two and a half, we felt as if the next member was ready to enter our family. Denise and I made love once a few days before she became fertile. This increased the likelihood of conceiving a daughter, as the female sperm was able to stay viable in the woman's reproductive system until the fertile egg was released. While Denise and I were breathing together that night, embraced in each other's loving arms, it felt like magic was rushing through us. Definitely a child conceived in pure love.

During the pregnancy, Denise listened to the Calm Birth practice often. I intended positive energy to the little one growing in my wife's womb. The birth happened about ten feet from where my mother delivered me, in the house that I grew up in. Denise was calm and focused. We held each other. I could feel this woman's strength. And sure enough, a little girl was born. Ivory came out with one arm reaching towards the sky. When she was only halfway out, she let out a little squawk, like to say, "Hey, look at me!"

Ivory quickly showed us she was going to be a strong woman that the world would have to deal with. She was calm in her crib. As soon as she could walk, she was off following her brother around the farm. When she fell, she would quickly yell at Denise and me, "I'm okay!" She has a confident strut that seems to say, "I know where I'm going."

The Calm Birth vase breathing meditation helped Denise and I develop and utilize our own innate skills as parents. We continue to use the practice to keep our parenting based in gratitude and positive intention to allow our children to grow into all they can be.

VII

Calm Mother Practices:
Empowering Postnatal Care

Even after their return home, most new mothers remain in partial seclusion with their babes for some length of time, sometimes glowing, sometimes trembling, as they absorb the impact of their experiences and try to integrate the new sets of meanings.

—Robbie E. Davis-Floyd[75]

So far, we've been focused on women's prenatal challenges and opportunities in the early twenty-first century. But today a woman's postnatal care concerns may be just as important. The problems with mind and anxiety that women may face postpartum can be disturbing, and may lead to chemical or other dependence. Postnatal practices to work with mind and anxiety may be as important to woman and infant health as prenatal mind-body methods. Such practices offer women means of self-empowerment after giving birth, through times often associated with anxiety and depression.

After years of development work on the Calm Birth prenatal practices, work began on a set of postnatal practices, for self-care, for child care, and for family care. The problems with postpartum depression and anxiety today may require strong medicine; and vase breathing, reclining progressive release, and compassionate breathing have proven that they can be that. The Calm Mother CD of postnatal meditation practices was released in 2006.

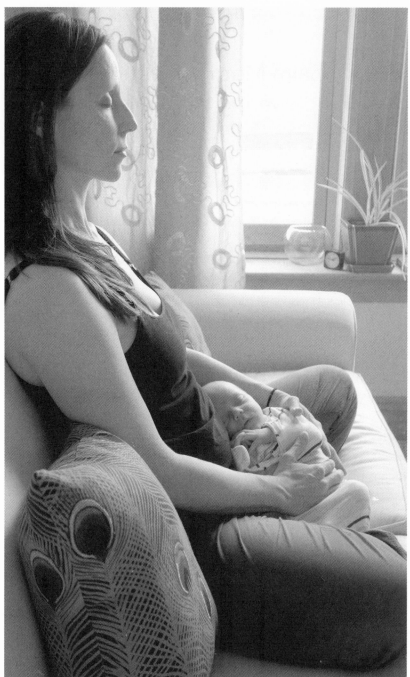

Eden meditating with her little one.

Photo by Judith Halek

Calm Mother Practice One: Calm Mother

Dr. Edmund Jacobson's groundbreaking work in neuromuscular release was further advanced in the medicine/meditation program at the University of Massachusetts Medical Center starting in 1979. Back in the 1930s and 1940s, the individual practicing one of Jacobson's progressive relaxation (PR) methods probably had some trouble maintaining focus, given the normal chaos of the mind; and yet, remarkably, Jacobson's PR self-care methods were consistently effective.

At UMMC, the application of mindfulness meditation to the practice of moment-by-moment neuromuscular release made the practice more efficient. Instead of randomly losing attention, the genius of mindfulness meditation enabled the person to maintain focus on the practice, resulting necessarily in more effective release, with a greater potential for healing the nervous system.

In the reclining meditation practice of Calm Mother, efficient neuromuscular release is applied to the aftermath of a labor and delivery process, whether it was a natural birth experience or not. Drugs, anesthesia, and surgery all challenge nervous system function.

Practicing the healing of her nervous system is as important for a woman after birth as it is in preparation for birth. The mother's healing is enhanced, and the child receives neural and other benefits through sympathetic resonance.

Another dimension of the Calm Mother progressive neuromuscular release in postnatal care is engagement with light on a cellular level. This builds vitality needed for recovery, extensive postnatal responsibilities, emotion, and disordered sleep. The postnatal experience of cellular light enhances the woman's sense of her body, for healthy self-respect and to regain deep reserves.

The Method

Following is a version of the audioguide transmission of the method.

The Practice (the audioguide, line by line)

This practice is done lying down.

It's a proven method to heal the nervous system.

It can free your nerves from the physical stress of birth.

This practice can also bring inner energy.

It can be a resource for years to come.

It's good for healing and regaining inner strength.

In this practice you go through your body

progressively releasing nervous tension.

You may increase life force

as you release disturbance and stress.

Find yourself a comfortable place to lie down.

You can lie down on your bed.

But if you lie on blankets on a rug,

or on a yoga mat and a blanket,

you'll probably be more alert and gain more from the practice.

You'll be able to have moment-by-moment release.

It's important to be comfortable and warm.

The effects are immediate

and they build over time.

The most benefits come from daily practice.

Lie down mindfully.

Please avoid falling asleep.

Keep your eyes open and soft.

This practice asks you to sense and enter

new dimensions,

so that you can realize more life.

It's good to close your eyes, from time to time,

but if you keep your eyes closed too much

you may tend to fall asleep.

To begin, take a deep breath,

and then exhale easily.

Feel the life energy working throughout your body.

Take another deep breath, deep into life,

and breathe out release for greater function.

As if you're doing it for the first time

be your whole vibrant body of life.

Feel the trillions of cells and the energy flows.

Let yourself feel the dynamic of all your systems.

There's so much life in you, it's inconceivable:

ten trillion living cells,

all working together for life.

When you feel your whole body directly,

you feel its unlimited life.

Keep feeling the sensation of all the pulsing currents,

the billionfold electric body process.

Feel all the life going on in you at once.

Feel yourself start to come all alive.

As you become aware of life itself in you,

if there's any discomfort or pain

let go of that. Let it unfold.

Let it flow out.

See how you tend to hold onto tension.

See how you can let it all go.

Let go of any stress or disturbance.

You're going to take this time to relax deeply,

all the way, slowly but surely.

Soon you'll go through your body

releasing tension, feeling your energy increase.

You'll release muscle tension on your nerves.

You do that with internal life support,

from the crown of your head to your feet.

Now starting with the toes of your feet,

feel all the life in your toes.

It's surprising how alive they are.

Feel the electric life in their bones.

Feel the energy channels running in your feet.

Feel their electric muscles and nerves.

Feel how it all works together.

Relax the muscles, tendons, and nerves in your feet.

Feel the service they have given you all these years.

Relax your feet into their open state.

Feel how this benefits your nerves.

Bring your attention from your feet

up through your ankles, into your calves.

Feel the energy running in and through them,

to and from all parts of your body.

Feel the life in the interconnection.

Find any tight muscles or tendons in your calves.

Relax the flesh into its great activity.

Feel the goodness of the electric flow,

the goodness of the blood flow,

the connection with the billionfold flows in your body.

Feel the depth of connection.

Feel the deep dimensions of your life support.

Come up from your calves into your knees.

Feel life force in your knees.

This is a good way to meditate,

appreciating living systems in your body,

releasing stress on your nerves.

You gain force as you release,

finding greater function.

Come up into your thighs.

Feel how they support your body.

Feel their muscles and nerves.

Optimize the aliveness of your flesh and bone.

Feel the muscles, nerves, and blood flow

throughout your hips and buttocks.

Notice any unnecessary tension.

Please soften it. Rest it all.

Release tensions and free your nerves.

Unlock and unblock, taking care of your own needs,

to have more to give.

Release any nerve restrictions.

Come into the basis of new life.

Bring your attention into your belly.

Sense if it holds any tension.

Please breathe down,

and let any anxiety go.

You can relax into greater life.

Now is the time to help yourself heal from any birth-related

surgery or disturbance.

You can finish with that now.

Come into greater function.

Feel your womb and all your inner female organs.

If there's any energy of disturbance there from the birth,

you can practice healing it now.

Let that release.

Sense all the fine tissue there and the nerves.

Breathe deeply into your womb, exhaling easily.

Bless and heal whatever needs to be healed.

Feel all the forces of life nourishing and sustaining you.

Intend blessing and sustenance into your female organs.

Feel how that tissue is sacred.

You're made to have that experience.

Place your hands lightly on your belly.

Touch your sense of the sacred with your hands.

Feel life force run in your arms and hands.

Feel your healing ability in your fingers.

Feel how much life you have to give.

Feel how much care and grace you have to give.

Feel whole and healed in yourself as the source of life.

Rest in your radiance and grace.

Now bring your attention into your spine.

Let your spine release and extend.

Feel the bones align.

Now feel your muscles throughout your rib cage and chest.

Release any tension there.

Let the muscles in your chest be free.

Feel your breasts alive with milk.

Feel the nourishment and gift in your milk.

Now feel the power of your heart.

Feel your heart beat for you and your child.

Feel it sustain your lives.

Pulse in the grace of that.

Bring your attention to your upper back, shoulders, and neck.

Stress and tension tend to be held there.

Breathe into that crucial area

and relax any accumulated tension.

Take your time.

Let the tension melt away.

Let your self be naturally free of stress.

Bring your attention into your face.

Feel your jaw and your mouth.

Let your lower face relax.

Let it rest.

Feel all the muscles around your mouth,

forming your conscious and unconscious expression.

Let all your expression there release.

Feel your mouth become free.

Bring your attention up to your eyes.

Feel all the muscles around them,

holding conscious and unconscious expression of your life.

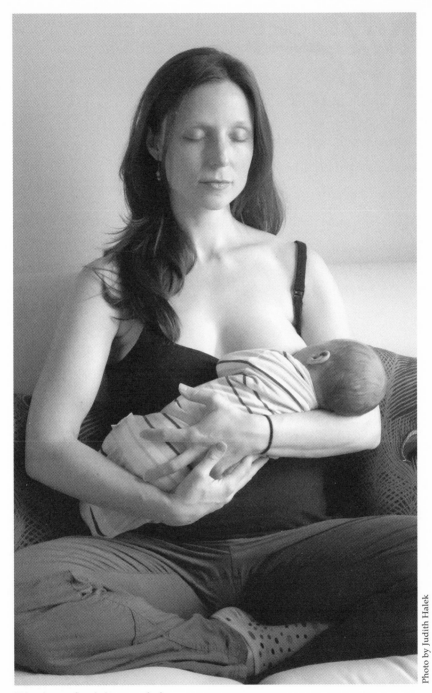

Eden breastfeeds her new baby.

Photo by Judith Halek

Relax all that completely. Let it go.

Let your face become completely free.

Feel your awareness come alive.

Feel the depth of your calm.

Resting in soft open eyes,

your energized body brims with life.

After giving birth you are reborn.

You receive more life beat by beat.

You feel your deep reserves.

As you finish the practice and start to arise,

lift yourself all alive.

Prepare to receive and give life as you move.

Calm Mother Practice Two: Sitting into Energy Body

Sitting into Energy Body is a sitting meditation in which the physical body and the energy body breathe together. This practice is from Tibet. You practice breathing vital energy from the air for greater function. In the postnatal period, a practice like Sitting into Energy Body can be empowering. For most women, postnatal meditation can be healing.

Visualization

There are two visualization concerns in this practice: what breathes, and what is breathed. Both require a more complete sense of the potential of human breathing and the life field in which the body breathes. Concerning what breathes, for most people it is a revelation that our bodies were made to breathe energy as well as oxygen. We are made to breathe vital energy from the air into a luminous breathing vase in the navel center of our energy system. The human body has millions of energy channels, but for the practice of Sitting into Energy Body we visualize just our central energy channel with its bright power centers, rising from the soft radiant Life Vase in our navel.

With respect to what is breathed, we visualize that what we call air is a field alive with universal energies. In it is vital energy fundamental to everything alive. It has been called universal chi, or prana, a subtle, life-giving substance. It has an affinity for the human body chi.

The Practice (the audioguide, line by line)

By sitting to calm and go deep,

you can transform breathing and mind.

You can practice energy breathing after giving birth.

You can breathe energy into your energy system. After giving birth, you can practice self-empowerment.

You can breathe energy into your Vase of Life.

In the beginning it's best to do this sitting practice

with audioguidance.

The audioguide practice takes twenty-three minutes.

Please use the CD or the MP3 files.

Each time the instructions become clearer.

Even when you know the instructions by heart

it's still good to practice at least twenty minutes a session,

and it's best to practice early in the day.

You can sit to reach deep resource to start the day.

You sit into vital energy systems to breathe completely.

Then throughout the day it's best to sit down

and regain the practice, for a few minutes each time.

If you sit and stop the world,

stopping to breathe energy into your energy system,

your body will take up the practice instinctively.

More and more the practice will come to you from the inside.

The more you do the practice,

the more you'll realize your energy system potential.

So sit down into your body to shift into your strength.

Sit to calm and breathe in a deeper way.

Sit on a cushion on the floor

or sit in a chair, upright and at ease.

Effortlessly balance your spine,

so that it naturally lifts a little.

Feel your stability and depth.

Now visualize your body in a deeper way.

See that inside your body is a body of energy channels.

Focus on the brilliant central energy channel,

from the crown of your head down to your navel.

At the bottom of the great channel, in your navel,

is the Vase of Life, a soft, luminous, breathing Vase

from which the central channel rises.

The Vase is there for you to bring energy into your body.

You breathe energy from the air into the Vase.

From the Vase, the energy rises up the central energy channel,

to feed your higher systems,

for you to start to realize your potential.

Many, many people have done this practice,

for centuries,

breathing energy from the air into the Vase of Life,

to come alive with greater function.

Please sit and breathe this way.

Sense the vital energy in the air.

It's always been there.

It's the universal energy that makes everything alive.

You were born to breathe vital energy in the air.

That energy is the basis of your life.

Begin by sensing life-giving energy in the air,

energy you've been breathing in and out without knowing.

Sense that you were made to breathe it into the Vase,

the soft, radiant Life Vase at the bottom of your central channel.

Now breathe in the life-giving energy intentionally

and direct it down into the Vase.

When you do, you'll feel it go into the Vase.

Easily breathe life-giving energy into your Vase of Life.

Please do it now.

Sense your physical and subtle body deeply.

Feel life sensation throughout.

Feel and see the breathing Vase in your navel center.

Breathe in and intend the vital energy from the air into your Vase.

Feel that you're breathing life energy down to your womb.

Feel how you're doing this to heal

whatever may need to be healed from the birth.

Breathe energy into the Life Vase near your womb.

As you sit and breathe in this deeper way, this healthier way,

breathing and intending vital energy down into the Life Vase,

your mind tends to distract you.

Instead of breathing vital energy for greater function,

you may find yourself lost in thought,

thinking about something that happened

or something you think is going to happen.

You're distracted.

Then something in you wants to wake up.

Something in you always wants to wake up.

Something in you free of your mind

wakes you up and brings you back.

Your awareness interrupts your mind and brings you back.

Come back to energy breathing.

Come back to breathing with your energy body.

Dispel your distractions.

Empower yourself after giving birth.

Breathe energy into the Vase of Life.

Breathe awareness of the greatness of the field of life.

Please do that now.

Sense and breathe the vibrant universal field again and again,

the vital field that constantly gives you life.

Sense that you can breathe that from the air.

Sense that you can breathe that into yourself.

This energy is given to you to use.

You can breathe it in and use your body in a new way.

You can live in a greater way after giving birth.

You're doing what is right and good for you to do.

Breathe in a greater way.

Breathe oxygen and vital energy.

You'll be more alive.

Breathe life from the air into your Vase with ease.

Your mind may interfere,

but your awareness is free of your mind.

Breathe with awareness, free of mind.

You'll start to know your mind.

You've been giving your power to your mind all your life.

This is the time for revolution.

Shift your power from your mind to your awareness.

Breathe vital energy with awareness.

Your mind will try to distract you.

The more you practice breathing life energy,

the more awareness you have,

the more you can see.

Breathe life into your Vase and have more life,

for your child, for your family, for the world.

Breathe to shift power to come alive.

Please breathe easily into the Vase.

Sometimes you'll wake up in the morning breathing this way.

You'll sit down into the calm that comes

with breathing completely.

You'll sit down into quiet energy.

In that quiet is the stillness of a higher order.

Breathe into energy body for greater life.

You can go to sleep this way.

Sit and calm into greater function.

Establish breathing into the Vase.

Raise the intention to breathe vital energy in your sleep.

Your unconscious mind can breathe energy in your sleep.

It can give you a deeper kind of rest.

You can rest, relaxing into greater function.

Then you may awake in a new way.

Breathe into a different kind of life.

Practice revolution into grace.

Shift your attention from your mind to your awareness.

Practice breathing life-giving energy in the air.

Please do that now.

Receive the life-giving energy field that makes the world alive.

Use the energy you were born to use.

Breathe life into your life,

and your child will touch greater life too,

in sympathetic resonance with you.

Please do this practice for yourself and others.

Please continue breathing effortlessly into the Vase.

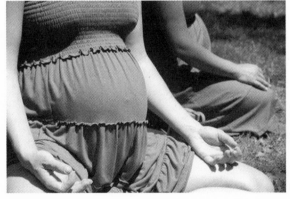

Photo by Judith Halek

VIII
New Childbirth Medicine

The new vision of the psyche has far-reaching implications not only for each of us as individuals but for professionals in psychology and medicine.

—Stanislav Grof[76]

Meditation and the Nature of the Child

Though the practices that Calm Birth is based on have been respected for a long time, their application in childbirth is new childbirth medicine. They are strong mind-body medicines.

Womb Breathing is both energy medicine and mind-body medicine. It works by breathing vital energy into the energy system and by shifting from mind to awareness, a dual means of improving childbirth health. The application of progressive neuromuscular release (Practice of Opening) to prenatal care may be the most important use of that proven mind-body medicine to date.

In prenatal meditation, pregnant women repeatedly shift their attention from mind to awareness, returning again and again to the innate awareness they're endowed with. They sense the innate awareness their wombchild is endowed with. And if we look into the nature of the child to see what is innate, meditation asks us to see that the inborn awareness is primal, primordial, and fundamental to the embryo. It's an early telepathic resource for the developing human.[77]

The woman's prenatal meditation may help the child maintain awareness as it is born, an important basis of psychophysical health.

A pregnant woman's prenatal meditation may inspire the child to be free of fear and have fearless confidence in awareness. Children may have stressful experiences during pregnancy and delivery. The resource of the woman's prenatal meditation serves as a reference point for the child to return to his or her own calming connection with innate awareness.

When the mother practices postnatal meditation, the child is again reminded of its innate awareness, a key to health, survival, and meaningful engagement with life. Such children may have an inclination to meditate as a foundation of their personal development.

New childbirth medicine gives us a vision of the potential of women's health in pregnancy and of the health of a child's awareness.

Benefits of Prenatal Audioguidance

All the research cited below concerning hearing in the womb is from the work of David Chamberlain:

> Signs of ear development can be seen in your prenate only a week after conception. By the halfway mark of pregnancy, elaborate labyrinths, chambers, and passageways with impressive nerve and brain connections are in place ... Since other parts of the baby's brain and nervous system are only partially insulated at birth, it seems that hearing has a very high priority.[78]

The womb is a dynamic sound chamber in which the infant is constantly hearing, responding to the sounds of the woman's body and to external sounds, which it perceives directly. The infant is particularly sensitive to the sound of the mother's voice. Her words, her songs, her sighs, her laughs reverberate throughout her body. Sound is transmitted remarkably well through the liquid crystal matrix of her flesh. The sound is louder and clearer than we might imagine. The infant may also hear through bone conduction.

For the pregnant woman practicing with the meditative sound of the audioguide, prenatal audioguidance may help neutralize negative conditioning for her and her child inseparably.

Some words heard during the pregnancy, including words the mother is listening to carefully, again and again, can inspire a higher level of attention in the wombchild. This may result in more advanced language skills in the child.

> Appropriate audio therapy in the perinatal period can positively influence the state of consciousness and protect from an inappropriate stress response. This gives us an opportunity to impart our love as well as our wisdom. The implications are that these modalities will lead to physical and emotional benefits to the mother and newborn as well as medical cost savings.[79]

The wombchild with the experience of prenatal audioguidance will be energetically in sympathetic resonance with its mother's attention to that voice, and it will hear that voice directly. That child can be born with inclinations to hear what others are saying, which would be an advantage in developing language and communication skills.

Advances in audio technology make it possible to hear the recorded human voice more clearly than it's ever been heard. With the Calm Birth prenatal practices CD, attention is engaged by the voice of meditation instruction with more impact than has been possible before. The voice of guidance can be heard vividly by woman and wombchild, a voice imparting a high level of childbirth care.

Paranormal Childbirth Experience

Many books and papers have been published about normal people having paranormal experiences, experiences of great ability and realization. Many of the reported paranormal experiences occur in near-death situations, where people experience being all-knowing, all-seeing, having marvelous powers, being full of unforgettable transformation.

Books have also been written researching paranormal childbirth experience. Some women have experiences of precognition or clairvoyance and have remarkable states of illumination in pregnancy and childbirth. With mind-body childbirth practice, there is a dual increase

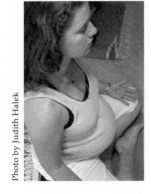

Photo by Judith Halek

in the potential for extraordinary experience, in the woman and in the child. Prenatal meditation methods, and natural childbirth in general, help women avoid unnecessarily medicated birth that limits the potential of awareness and realization. Even in the face of medical intervention, though, childbirth meditation offers woman and child ways to more fully access the great human experience potential of childbirth.

Regarding childbirth offering paranormal potential, Danah Zohar, celebrated MIT and Harvard professor of physics and philosophy, now at Oxford, writes:

> During the pregnancy of my first child, and for some months after her birth, I experienced what for me was a strange new way of being. In many ways I lost the sense of myself as an individual, while at the same time gaining a sense of myself as part of some larger and ongoing process ... At first the boundaries of my body extended inwards to embrace and become one with the new life growing inside me. I felt complete and self-contained, a macrocosm within which all life was enfolded ... During those months, "I" seemed a very vague thing, something on which I could not focus or get a grip, and yet I experienced myself as extending in all directions, backwards into "before time" and forwards into "all time," inwards toward all possibility and outwards towards all existence ...[80]

Elisabeth Hallett, researcher in paranormal birth experiences, published the account of a woman who reports the following:

> I had gone to sleep feeling very peaceful and comfortable with my pregnancy; almost in a meditation state. Upon waking, the clearest dream-vision was overpowering in my memory. I was seeing through my son's bright blue eyes—his hands drifting through the pale fluid. Then I was seeing his face. Large blue eyes; almost translucent skin, ears, nose, eyelids ...[81]

This kind of experience is explicitly encouraged by Practice of Opening.

Practice of Opening may enable paranormal childbirth experience for some people. This practice encourages extraordinary seeing and knowing. It can help women to see on a cellular level and know life force directly, and it can enable direct communication with the womb-child. Womb Breathing encourages recognition and use of energy systems designed for action beyond ordinary ranges of activity. Giving and Receiving helps women recognize and use their ability to transform their sense of body, in childbirth and beyond.

It would be healthy for this planet if near-birth experiences came to be considered as important a part of the legend of human life as near-death experiences.

Empathic Childbirth Medicine

A pregnant woman sits in effortless meditation. The image of a pregnant woman sitting in meditation is remarkably similar to a buddha statue. The double form of it is profound: a buddha with a buddha within. The woman has taken the posture of physical and psychological stability and balance for two lives at once. The sitting meditation form of a pregnant woman is one of sitting to have a psychologically and physically undisturbed birth. It's an empathic form. It's a form of care.

Ashley Montagu's book *The Natural Superiority of Women* (1954) envisioned that superiority in terms of a compassionate nature. *Webster's New World College Dictionary* (1986) defines the word "humane" as "having what are considered the best qualities of human beings; kind, tender, merciful, sympathetic, etc.; civilizing; humanizing." The pregnant woman practicing sitting meditation is a form of humane being. She practices empathic care.

Meditation Science and Medical Science

Characteristics of the various kinds of meditation available from different meditation traditions in the West vary substantially, but the published results of extensive studies and books clearly indicate a wide range of meditation benefits for each method. The first meditation studies employed Transcendental Meditation, a mantra-based technique. The first studies of the meditation's impact on melatonin levels employed mindfulness meditation, a psychological method. Further research would probably show that each method produces elevated levels of both hormones.

Practice of Opening should tend to yield results similar to those observed in Jacobson's work and in the UMMC program, but the

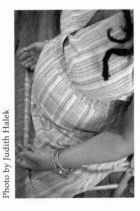

Photo by Judith Halek

Practice of Opening audioguidance language was developed to produce new maternal and infant benefits.

Similarly, the practice of Womb Breathing should bring benefits similar to those extensively observed in Buddhist mindfulness practice; yet, Womb Breathing has complete breathing, energy breathing, which gives the practice an additional biophysical domain. Though based on the traditional practice of vase breathing, Womb Breathing was adapted for the needs of childbirth medicine. The additional benefits of Womb Breathing need to be observed. Research protocols are being prepared.

The practice of Giving and Receiving is based on the Buddhist practice of *ton len,* proven effective for centuries and now used in various healing applications. Though ton len is being researched in the West, given the potential for healing in pregnancy, the childbirth application of ton len should be researched. One intention of this book is to draw interest and support for research in mind-body childbirth practices in general.

For medical science to evaluate the benefits of prenatal meditation, it must appreciate the foundation of meditation in proven science, "deep science."[82] Ken Wilber says:

> Where the exemplar in the physical sciences might be a telescope, and in the mental sciences might be linguistic interpretation, in the

spiritual sciences the exemplar, the injunction, the paradigm, the practice is: meditation or contemplation. It too has its injunctions, its illuminations, and its confirmations, all of which are repeatable—verifiable or falsifiable—and all of which therefore constitute a perfectly valid mode of knowledge acquisition.[83]

Contemporary EEG studies of meditative states, continues Wilber, show that meditation

... produces dramatic and repeatable changes in the entire organism, and most significantly in the electrical patterns of the brain itself, presumably the seat of consciousness... To check or refute the claims of meditation science, investigators will have to use deep science: namely, take up the injunction or paradigm of meditation; gather the data, the direct experience.[84]

In other words, to experience something of the potential of the use of mind-body practice in pre- and postnatal care, you'd have to first experience meditation directly.

IX

The Evolution of Mind-Body Practice in Obstetrics

I personally believe that subtle energy medicine is on the verge of scientific breakthroughs that alone could revolutionize the objective dimensions of medical care.

—Ken Wilber[85]

In order to look at the history and potential of mind-body practice in obstetrics, we have to look at the shift of medical practice in general. Larry Dossey, MD, has given us a good model for that shift. He sees that three eras of medicine (as described in the "Emerging Possibilities" section of the Preface) have evolved and are present all at once—physical medicine, mind-body medicine, and transpersonal medicine. The emergence of mind-body medicine in obstetrics began with the use of hypnosis in France from the 1880s on to relieve women of labor pain. Clinical hypnosuggestive therapy is like physical medicine in that it keeps the patient passive. It is unlike physical medicine in that it helps the patient's mind act as an analgesic agent.

The next stage in the evolution of mind-body practice in obstetrics is a leap to self-applied mind-body practice: the psychoprophylactic method (key date 1951). It is based on preparation through education in natural childbirth, with the Pavlovian focus on language as a physiological trigger. Like hypnosis, it is based on the psychology of dissociation.[86] Patterned breathing is used as a distraction from pain.

The third stage in the evolution of mind-body practice in obstetrics is another leap, to the more complete model of the woman's body and potential. It's founded on more than a thousand years of meditation science and more than forty years of the practice of mind-body medicine in America. The third stage of mind-body practice in obstetrics is founded on the meditation-based pain management program of the University of Massachusetts Medical Center, from 1979 to the present, and it is also based on advances in subtle energy medicine. Stage 3 mind-body obstetrics practice works with the integral union of the physical body, the psychosomatic body, and the energy body. A Stage 3 obstetrician respects traditional medical knowledge of the energy body and its power centers.[87] Stage 3 mind-body practice helps prevent suffering in childbirth through recognition and release of anxiety and fear, with the biological enrichment of complete breathing and greater function.

In all three stages of mind-body practice in obstetrics, pain is subject to the influence of the spoken and/or written word. Stage 3 practices may also give freedom from mind and words and entrance into the full potential of the woman's body and awareness in childbirth. This integral model of childbirth offers a more open and courageous psychology, probably with more potential for human health and development than in the earlier stages of mind-body practice in obstetrics.

Stage 1: Hypnosis

Hypnosis is a distinctive, often trance-like mental state that is induced by an organized pattern of suggestions, usually verbal in nature, beginning with the suggestion of relaxation. The suggestions may be directly induced by a hypnotist in the presence of the subject, but may also be self-induced (self-hypnosis or autohypnosis/auto-suggestion).[88] The word "hypnosis" itself is the invention of nineteenth-century Scottish physician James Braid. Although the long-held popular view was that hypnosis is a form of unconsciousness, the informed contemporary view is that it is actually a wakeful state of focused attention and heightened suggestibility,[89] with diminished peripheral awareness.[90] As defined in Goleman and Gurin's *Mind-Body Medicine*,[91] hypnosis is a form of induced, focused attention that can make it easier for a person to control mind-body functions.

Background

Though Franz Mesmer's controversial demonstrations of "animal magnetism" as a psychotherapeutic agent in Paris were not successful,[92] he did significantly influence others to explore working with patients psychotherapeutically, inducing medically valuable states.

Charles Lafontaine (1803–92), a mesmerist, made a dramatic demonstration of mind-body influence through suggestion in London in 1841. It strongly influenced neurosurgeon James Braid, who was in the audience. Within a year, Braid made his own inspired use of the mesmerist method, defining a new psychotherapeutic agent, hypnosis, and a new therapeutic field, hypnotherapy.[93] His method required repose and general quietude to induce a state of somnolence, a state of "brain and central nervous system mobility."[94] Braid saw that physiology could be influenced therapeutically through the mind. As a medical doctor, he sensed the far-reaching potential of hypnotically induced mind-body effects in medicine, especially for pain management.

Braid had several significant French medical doctor disciples, including Étienne Eugène Azam (1822–99) of Bordeaux; Pierre Paul Broca (1824–80), an anatomist; the physiologist Joseph-Pierre Durand de Gros (1826–1900); and the eminent hypnotist, cofounder of the Nancy School, Ambroise-Auguste Liébeault (1823–1904). Fernand Lamaze said that by

> 1880 French physicians were known to be using hypnosis as a therapeutic agent at the Salpêtrière Hospital in Paris; so had Bernheim in Nancy… They pointed out that it was possible to use it to induce a state of insensitivity that allowed operations to be performed.[95]

Essential to the therapeutic use of hypnosis was and is the mind-body effect, requiring the patient's focused attention and will, whether induced by a doctor or self-induced. As we shall see, clinical hypnotic induction and guided meditation have similar effects, and as the use of mind-body methodology in OB has advanced, the principles of self-hypnotic induction and guided meditation are valuable to that advance.

The Use of Hypnosis in Obstetrics

In 1899, Paul Joire, OB/GYN, of Lille, France, made remarkable break-throughs in the application of hypnosis to manage pain in child-birth. He demonstrated importantly that pain and contractions are not related. The experience of pain comes after the sensation of con-traction. He was aware of the technical difficulties of hypnosis and favored the use of suggestion in the fully conscious pregnant woman. He explained the natural function of contractions, saying that there was no need for the experience of pain, that pain was neither nec-essary nor helpful. He gave women a means to participate in and consciously influence the quality of the birth.

The center of research into the use of hypnosis in obstetrics shifted to the USSR after the revolution in 1917. With a national health pro-gram based on the Nobel Prize science of Ivan Pavlov (1849–1936), physiologist and psychologist, some Soviet obstetricians applied hyp-nosis in childbirth through the 1920s and 1930s, on into the 1940s. The USSR was poor and there were shortages of medicine. There was a mass pain management problem. The goal of the use of hypnotherapy in childbirth was to evolve a psychotherapeutic obstetrics technique to reduce or eliminate the need for costly nitrous oxide, novocaine, morphine, ether, and chloroform. After the decimation of the Russian population in World War II, women were widely encouraged to have children, and the government wanted to make childbirth appealing to them. Soviet obstetrics wanted to offer women "painless childbirth" with little or no medicine. In the severity of their shortages, they needed to offer significant psychotherapeutic alternatives.

In 1923 Platonov and Velvovsky presented their report on hypno-suggestive analgesia to the Second Pan-Russian Congress of Psychia-trists and Neurologists, describing uses of hypnosuggestive analgesia in surgery, obstetrics, and gynecology. However, it was left to Nico-laiev, in 1927, to pioneer the application of hypnosis in obstetrics in the light of Pavlov's theories, and it was from that date that he and Platonov clearly demonstrated the importance of "fighting fear in the woman by means of a psychotherapeutic approach."[96]

Several methods were explored. Some women were induced into a state of hypnotic sleep at the time of delivery. Others were prepared in a state of hypnosis but brought back to consciousness for the birth. The clinician chose whether or not to be present the whole time. Indirect suggestion was also applied. An anesthetic mask was used, but no gas was made to flow through it. Some women using autosuggestion were fully awake.[97]

However, the clinical application of hypnosis in obstetrics in the USSR did not evolve to be the "universal" mind-body method that was desired. In the 1940s there was increasing dissatisfaction with the variance of the quality of ability in the medical practitioners and variance in the receptiveness of patients. Clinical capability in hypnotherapy required intensive training, and then it was time-consuming for the obstetrician in practice. It concentrated on the symptomatic treatment of pain over a period of hours and sometimes longer. It also encouraged passivity in the woman, which was not desirable. Finally, it was found to be of limited help with the real causes of pain. Countersuggestions from the woman's environment and upbringing could nullify the efforts of the obstetrician.

There was progress in the development of other mind-body methods in the USSR in the late 1940s, and among them the psychoprophylactic method emerged to become the official childbirth method in the USSR and a significant achievement for the mind-body method in obstetrics.

Stage 2: The Psychoprophylactic Method

Behind the use of hypnosis in obstetrics in the USSR was the inspiration of Pavlovian science concerning the neurology and physiology of conditioned reflexes. Having observed that responses are conditioned, we can observe that we can change conditioning. In the field of medicine, the idea of changing conditioned responses to pain, particularly in childbirth, required a shift to self-care, where education was essential. Education in the nature of the human pain experience and in the physical facts of childbirth was essential to changing conditioned responses in childbirth.

Instead of hypnosis and suggestion that concentrated on the symptomatic treatment of pain, Velvovsky recommended a preventive training of the fully conscious woman by means of educational methods. This approach appealed to the perceptive faculties of the woman, and encouraged her to take an active part in her delivery, which remained under her control.[98]

In 1933, Platonov published his book *The Spoken Word as a Physiological and Therapeutic Agent.* The ultimate aim of Platonov and Velvovsky was to change the attitude of women and all of society toward the pain of childbirth.

As the Psychoprophylactic Method (PPM) program was being developed in a few clinics, childbirth preparation classes were attended once a week for six or eight weeks, and the woman was required to read the literature and practice patterned breathing exercises at home. The program emphasized deep breathing, but "… over time the number of breathing patterns recommended for different stages of labor became quite complex and cumbersome."[99]

The term "psychoprophylaxis" was first presented by Nicolaiev in 1949. Later that year, in Kharkov, in the Ukraine, Velvovsky, Platonov, and their associates demonstrated and defined PPM. In 1951, in a major declaration of Soviet health care policy, it was mandated that PPM be applied in every normal birth in all birthing establishments throughout the USSR. They needed to package it quickly for vast dissemination, and then try to evaluate outcomes. Communication was slow then.

Fernand Lamaze, an OB/GYN practicing in Paris, had been keenly interested in the development of mind-body obstetrics techniques in the USSR. He was there in 1951 for the historic mandate. He had trouble being allowed to witness a demonstration of the method; but when he did, he was very impressed. He said that as a sixty-year-old obstetrician, he felt like a little boy compared to the level of the Soviet psychotherapist obstetricians he met. He completely believed that the program was effective and well defined. He was satisfied with it as a demonstration of Pavlovian science in childbirth.

Lamaze had founded his obstetrics practice in Paris in 1947 at the Maternité du Métallurgiste. That means that he was the obstetrician at the obstetrics clinic of the pro-communist metal workers union. Lamaze idealized the USSR. He agreed to present PPM in the West exactly as it was taught in the USSR. When he returned from the USSR in 1951, inspired to apply the Soviet childbirth method in the West, he did so in a field of extremely serious Cold War tensions, where his extolling of Soviet methods offended many French people.

PPM was implemented in the USSR at a time of national poverty and high anxiety. When we speak of the power of the spoken or written word to influence conditioning, we have to sense how life was in Stalinist USSR, with widespread fear caused in part by all the violence it took to form the totalitarian state through two world wars. The words spoken by the obstetricians and midwives carried the voice of the authority of the totalitarian state. All women everywhere in the USSR were required to use one method for normal births, using patterned breathing to distract and dissociate from labor pain.[100] It was applied for low expense and ease of training.

Though the Soviets and Lamaze proclaimed great success for PPM, today the Soviet evaluation methods appear clearly inadequate. One of the keys to the failure of PPM lies in the translation of the word "psychoprophylactic" itself. It is widely called "painless childbirth." We note that part of applying Pavlovian principles to childbirth was the belief by Soviet psychotherapists that they could psychologically "destroy" and "eradicate" pain from the childbirth experience. For them and for Lamaze, pain was negative. If a woman moaned or writhed during labor, the Soviet doctors disapproved, often making a negative tongue-clicking sound, making the birth more stressful for the woman. But denial and propaganda heralded the method.[101]

The Soviet government's voice was loud and clear, and women's voices were almost mute. The Soviet and Lamaze PPM was promoted as a method of liberating women, but for many women it was the opposite. With the Lamaze method, "the woman actually colludes in her own denial by adopting a system that 'controls' her response to pain, her breathing, her position, and even the sounds she makes, the most basic aspects of a laboring woman's behavior."[102]

Lamaze called PPM a "physiological and experimental method aimed … at abolishing pain associated with uterine contraction."[103] Note serious concerns here: The breathing exercises that Soviet OB doctors and Lamaze implemented were, to use Lamaze's terminology, "experimental." That is: as far as we know, none of the PPM obstetricians were trained in the sciences of breathing available in traditional medicine. (This is in sharp contrast to Stage 3 obstetrics methodology, which is based on profound knowledge of breathing.)

Today we can see that PPM didn't distinguish enough between the experiences of pain, fear, and suffering, between the normal sensation of labor contractions and what the mind may do in response. But it was a great event in the evolution of mind-body practice in obstetrics; and hundreds of thousands of women in the USSR, in China, and in the West experienced successful natural childbirths with the method, though even more may have experienced failure because they couldn't dissociate from the normal intensity of contractions. There also has been a concern over maternal fatigue and the possibility of hyperventilation from the use of the rapid, shallow pant-breaths during labor.[104]

Stage 3: Prenatal Meditation

The use of mind-body practice in obstetrics is presently proceeding mainly through the use of meditation in childbirth preparation. This includes prenatal yoga programs. In Stage 3, teaching women obstetrics meditation can help them to self-initiate into new levels of childbirth capability.

The shift from Stage 1 mind-body obstetrics practice to Stage 2 was a transition from doctor-controlled health care, where the woman was mostly passive and submissive, to self-care, where the woman was actively involved in the outcome of the birth. Stage 3 has emerged from our need for a complete model of the woman's body and potential in childbirth. Stage 3 mind-body obstetrics practice expands and deepens our sense of what the woman's mind-body is. It gives us the physical body, the quantum physics body, and the energy body in one. It's supported by various living traditions of meditation science and by a remarkable amount of contemporary clinical evidence. Stage 3 obstetrics mind-body practice is strongly supported by evidence-based medicine.

Stage 3 is founded on the pain and anxiety management program of the University of Massachusetts Medical Center (UMMC). That program has long proved that mindfulness meditation is a remarkable method of pain and anxiety management, using current scientific standards. Because more than twenty thousand people have taken the UMMC eight-week medicine/meditation program, and because clinical and research standards are higher now than at previous times in the history of medicine, it is possible to offer women scientifically respected mind-body practice for obstetrics.

Simultaneous with the UMMC program, meditation traditions have been a growing presence throughout the West. Increasing numbers of women are practicing meditation methods when they become pregnant. Childbirth preparation practice involving meditation is desirable to many pregnant women, those with meditation experience and those interested in learning.

In surveying the variety of meditation methods available for childbirth application, including advances in mind-body medicine made for childbirth, we have several methods available that are naturally complementary and can be described to indicate Stage 3 obstetrics practices:

» Mindfulness-based labor management
» Awareness-based energy breathing
» Progressive neuromuscular release

Mindfulness-Based Labor Management

The proving ground for meditation as a pain and anxiety management method has been all the people attending the UMMC program and the hundreds of other hospital Mindfulness-Based Stress Reduction programs it has generated, from 1979 to the present, in Canada and Europe as well as in the United States. Among those people have been thousands of patients with terminal cancer, critical cardiovascular problems, and irreparable nervous system damage. They have almost all been cases where the application of more medication or surgery would be dangerous, and where the pain levels were sometimes considered intolerable. "Extensive research conducted at UMMC demonstrated that meditation produced significant reductions in the following: present moment pain, negative body image, inhibition of activity, psychological disturbance, anxiety, and depression, and the need for pain-related drugs."[105] Inseparable from the significant pain management capability demonstrated by mindfulness meditation is its important anxiety management ability. Many medical and health care professionals participated in the program to learn an important method that has several potential uses.

Today mindfulness meditation is respected by the medical establishment as a practical tool, and we find mindful childbirth programs emerging,[106] very much based on the method as taught at UMMC.

The key to the function of mindfulness meditation in childbirth is the innate ability of the pregnant woman to distinguish between her mind and her awareness in order to recognize and release stress and anxiety. Because the woman is able to expose her mind to her awareness,[107] she is able to recognize incidents of anxiety and fear in herself without reacting, without being disturbed. The woman is able to have a psychologically undisturbed birth.

The preparation for mindfulness-based labor management is daily mindfulness practice, which becomes natural and ongoing. Edges of anxiety that may arise are met with patience and an inclination to calm down. Increased tolerance of pain is a developed disposition to not react to mind and emotion, allowing a state of openness and courage, with unrestricted physical and psychological function.

Awareness-Based Energy Breathing

The form of mindfulness practice described above is based on the Era I and Era II models of the woman's body: the physical and the mind-body models. Another form of mindfulness practice, awareness-based energy breathing, is based on the Era III model of the woman's body, the energy system model, and can integrate the best of the three eras of medicine.

All the characteristics of mindfulness meditation described above are equally true of awareness-based energy breathing. It uses exactly the same mindfulness technique but with an Era III model of the woman's body. Her inseparable physical body and energy body have different breathing capabilities. Women are endowed to breathe with both the energy body and the physical body at once.[108] With energy breathing, a pregnant woman may breathe completely to access full mind-body-spirit capability in labor.

Progressive Neuromuscular Release

From the very start of the UMMC medicine/meditation program in 1979, reclining progressive relaxation (PR), progressive neuromuscular release, was used as a complement to sitting mindfulness meditation. Jon Kabat-Zinn adapted Jacobson's whole-body practice for healing the nervous system (body scan), turning it into a reclining practice of mindfulness meditation, with increased attention to moment-by-moment neuromuscular release. In doing so, the UMMC method advanced PR as a therapeutic agent.

In applying the UMMC PR advancement to childbirth, there is a shift to the Era III model of the woman's body. In guided meditation, as the woman practices the progressive release of stresses on her nervous system, she practices healing her nervous system and her child's at the same time. She's connecting to her quantum body, a body of atomic light. She simultaneously practices shifting from mind to awareness while releasing neuromuscular stress. As she does so, she may discover life-supportive dimensions of her energy body, and she may experience developmental bonding with her wombchild.[109]

Comparing Stage 3 mind-body obstetrics practice with Stage 1, we can see that induction instructions given by OBs using hypnosis for pain management are comparable to the instructions of childbirth methods today that use guided imagery.[110] With respect to all three Stage 3 methods described above, today women have audioguides, made with sensitive voice intonations. Some give authentic prenatal and

189

postnatal meditation instruction. Women play the instruction CDs or MP3 files as a practice guide, but they must do the practices for themselves, consciously and silently. They are active, in a healthful way, compared with the passivity of birthing women in Stage 1 mind-body obstetrics practice and in medical birth.

Integral Childbirth Care

Imagine that we have the basis of a new childbirth health care system founded on integral medicine. The concept of integral medicine was defined in the 1940s from an older sense of the need for a total or complete model of patient care. When integral medicine is our model, body, mind, and spirit are inseparable. And Ken Wilber, in *Consciousness and Healing: Integral Approaches to Mind-Body Medicine*, says that the physician or care provider must be cared for, too. All factors that affect health must be considered.[111]

We can say that integral childbirth care began with Soviet/Lamaze PPM, educating women and teaching them a mind-body method that enabled them to be actively involved in the birth. That's healthier for the woman and child than ignorant and passive birth and may avoid the risks of medical birth. Prenatal meditation offers us a more complete model of care. Through the use of mind-body and energy meditation, we are evolving a more complete vision of the potential of maternal and infant health.

If complete childbirth care is to be given to women, they should be offered the model of complete function early in the pregnancy as a primary option, whether or not a medical birth is planned. The model of complete-function birth has the support of subtle energy science that exists in various traditions and the increasing scientific study of the human energy system. We can sense the importance of energy system care in childbirth and in women's health in general. The amount of care that a woman is actually given in childbirth depends on how completely her body is respected.

When a woman receives childbirth education in the Era III model of medicine, she learns how to use her energy system in comprehensive prenatal care. Integral childbirth means that if the pregnant woman is not offered mind-body and energy breathing practice, she is not receiving potentially important care that could help her significantly affect the quality of the pregnancy, the birth, and parenthood.

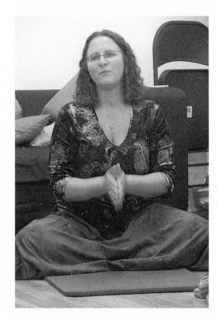
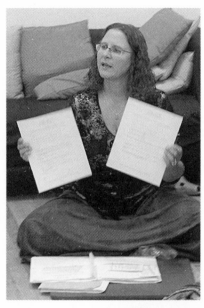

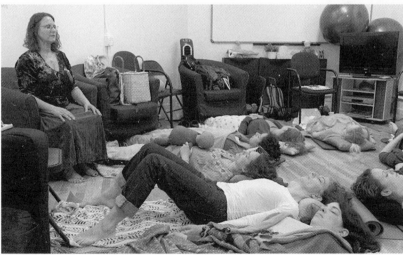

Photos by Judith Halek

Christine Novak, RNC-OB, conducting a Calm Birth teacher training, New York City, June 2010.

X

Toward a New Era of Childbirth Education

The human being, in essence, is in the process of discovering self-responsibility and personal empowerment. These two newly emerging characteristics contain the necessary seeds for creating an entirely new global society.

—Caroline Myss[112]

Both spontaneously and through transformational practice, a new evolutionary domain is rising in the human species.

—Michael Murphy[113]

Seen with new eyes, our lives can be transformed from accidents into adventures. We can transcend the old conditioning...We have new ways to be born.

—Marilyn Ferguson[114]

In childbirth medicine today, through the widespread use of anesthesia and pain-blocking chemicals, awareness is suppressed in the large majority of the births in the industrialized countries. Although the medical establishment may believe that the reduction or elimination of awareness of labor pain is a compassionate intervention, and though chemically induced calm may allow other interventions that make the process of childbirth convenient for doctors and lucrative for hospitals, the routine suppression of awareness in childbirth may be diminishing human quality. In the large majority of births, women do not function in the way they were made to, and most are unaware as that happens.

This is a pivotal concern for a needed revolution in childbirth education. Quality of awareness is a vital concern in childbirth. Suppression of awareness interferes with maternal and infant health. The recognition, cultivation, and protection of the prenatal awareness of the woman and child may be the most essential challenge to childbirth medicine today. The shift in the medical paradigm lets us see the problems deeply and lets us see and feel the need for great change in childbirth practice and education.

Establishing the Value of Awareness in Childbirth

Understanding that the awareness of the woman and of the womb-child are most often suppressed by prevalent labor interventions that have biological and psychological risks, we need to establish a new priority of respect for the awareness of the pregnant woman and the awareness of the child in the womb. Natural childbirth today is founded on prenatal awareness. Such programs empower women to remain aware, trust their innate capability, and make choices that will protect their right to give birth naturally. This supports their access to important developmental experiences, sometimes including extraordinary realization, while avoiding interventions that can reduce or take away that potential.

Preparation for the childbirth experience is an opportunity for both parents and prenates to communicate and develop psychologically. Natural childbirth training is not just about how to tolerate labor pain; it enables women to appreciate the intelligence of labor contractions and to come to greater awareness.[115] Various exercises, particularly breathing exercises, are offered in natural childbirth classes to preserve the integrity of awareness and natural capability.

Today, with the increasing availability of meditation methods in the West, more and more women come to pregnancy with a developed sense of the nature of awareness from meditation. Such women would almost certainly choose childbirth education in which meditation training was an important option, if it was available. With mind-body practices based on knowledge of complete breathing and greater function, we could be on the threshold of a new era of natural childbirth. Appropriate childbirth education, incorporating meditation science supported by more sensitive medical protocols, could offer women a new level of childbirth experience and health. That would be great for the prenates. The education pregnant women need can be founded on empowering self-care practices and a more complete model of the woman's body and potential. Though we have the knowledge and the methods, the medical establishment has resisted using them for decades. What can change this situation?

When the vast USSR was bankrupt after World War II, when it had very little money for medical birth—ether, chloroform, morphine, surgery—it mandated that all normal births had to use their "painless childbirth" mind-body program. Financial collapse, painful as that would be, may be beneficial for childbirth. The use of medical interventions would be minimized. Childbirth education would be transformed. Healthy mind-body and subtle energy methods would be used in the hospitals and homes. Proven methods already exist ready to be used.

Unproven methods are prevalent in the controversial current state of perinatal technologies, as malpractice lawsuits continue to increase. Meanwhile, the use of the word "science" in conjunction with the word "meditation" reflects the fact that several renowned meditation traditions are based on centuries of experience with highly refined methods and knowledge of their psychological and physiological consequences. Extensive literature exists, much of it in excellent translation now and accessible internationally, describing the methods and effects of these sciences. That literature is revered and is the basis of great teaching traditions. Buddhism has always called itself a science of human development rather than a religion. In its meditation science, psychological phenomena are observed from a basis of invaluable experience and sophisticated methodology. Meditation science has adhered to the deepest principles of science. In comparison, some of the most vaunted twentieth-century sciences, for lack of vision, have threatened this planet with the gravest of dangers, whereas meditation science has proved beneficial through the ages, doing no harm but much good.

And may women *empower themselves through* meditation in childbirth preparation for ages to come.

Change and Paradigm Shift

Let's consider changes taking place in the medical establishment that will make it possible to create a new quality of childbirth education and birth.

A reductionist form of medicine (also called material, mechanical, or physical medicine) has dominated medical practice for at least a hundred years.[116] This form of medicine holds tenaciously to the idea that human consciousness is a product of the brain.

From this limited perspective, the brain of a human fetus is considered incomplete, the brain of a newborn still immature, and intelligence or awareness is unexpected until months or years after birth. This justifies aggressive medical interventions during labor and delivery, during postpartum routines in hospital care, as well as during surgery at all phases, including intrauterine surgery, surgical delivery, and major surgery postpartum. In prevalent birth medicine, the wombchild is ignored. This means that doctors and nurses, however compassionate they may be as individuals, offer care constrained by accepted medical beliefs and values they were taught in school. It's convenient for medical birth to assume mistakenly that the wombchild is unaware. In fact, the child can be very aware.

Fortunately, in the last few decades, medical practice has been expanding its understanding of the infant senses, including the reality of infant pain perception, and has begun to consider that there might be levels of development that include emotion and thought associated with the infant brain.

Mind-body medicine offers a direct approach to the awareness of the wombchild, awareness that may be present remarkably early. Mind-body methods respect and encourage the child's prenatal intelligence.

Today there are educators who feel that it is crucial to incorporate new guidelines and values based on women's rights to appropriate education. There are educators and attorneys who see women's and infants' rights as essential concerns. What is too often missing in the current childbirth education curricula are the appreciation of awareness and of the low-risk, low-expense methods that bring natural, self-induced calm to the drama of childbirth.

Awareness and Life Itself

Adults and children can directly experience the timeless and open quality of awareness at any moment. Children can readily learn meditation. They have a knack for experiencing inherent open awareness. Prenates may have natural meditation. In prenatal psychology, the mental states of prenates have been tracked across the decades in measurements of memory and learning. As learning theories themselves became more sophisticated and testable, the evidence for learning in the womb became more dramatic and persuasive. The technology of heartbeat measurement was an early breakthrough, and the perfection of ultrasound made possible the study of fetal behavior in reaction to specific stimuli. Ultimately, a combination of such measurements made it possible to reveal learning in all periods of development in the womb. Similarly, depth memory work in various altered state therapies has demonstrated embryonic awareness of the feelings expressed by mothers and fathers at the discovery of their pregnancy.[117]

In sensing that universal awareness may be innate in the moment of human conception, innate in the embryo, we can sense the immanence of intelligent forces of great magnitude required to produce the embryo of a body designed to carry potentially unlimited awareness.

Thus, self-awareness is probably a *very* early experience of the fetus. Evidence of awareness and intelligence is being noted at earlier and earlier stages of development.[118] David Chamberlain says:

> Prenatal and perinatal memories are transpersonal in transcending all the expected boundaries of consciousness during intrauterine time and birth, especially memory, learning, sensation,

emotion, perception, thought, dreaming, out-of-body experience, near-death experience, clairvoyance, and telepathy. None of these phenomena of consciousness were anticipated in the materialistic paradigm of twentieth century developmental psychology. In fact they were rejected...[119]

In Chamberlain's important book, *Windows to the Womb: Revealing the Conscious Baby from Conception to Birth,* he is able to define twelve senses of the child in the womb, including telepathy. He speaks of the baby as having psychic rather than physiological vision. He finds that the "womb baby" has "primal consciousness" and may see beyond barriers with extrasensory perception. He says, "... babies in the womb can be seen plunging ahead using the intuitive and psychic powers that are their true birthright."[120]

The last chapter of Chamberlain's book is called "Conception and Before: Consciousness before Brain." To convey his sense of how extraordinary it is that awareness may well be present at conception, of how extraordinary a baby is, he sees that the womb baby's "consciousness is primal, formative, and overarching"[121] and not the product of a physical brain. He sees wisdom and empathy in the wombchild from the start of intrauterine life.

More scientists are agreeing with meditation teachers that awareness precedes and may create matter.

Knowledge and the Moment of Conception

I believe that the subject of reincarnation should be discussed in appropriate childbirth education. Below are some reasons why.

The human egg and sperm unite to form the zygote, millions and millions of living molecules, all of them vitalized by powerful atoms. Inside the atomic function of the zygote are space and electric force. Inside the atomic space is the universal quantum field, the universal potential, probably completely aware. The zygote may carry some momentum of reincarnation. The key may be in the nature of inherent primal awareness, free of mind yet carrying traces of the past.

Stan Grof says in his book *The Holotropic Mind:*

> Research in transpersonal psychology continues to provide ample evidence that this area of study [reincarnation] is a veritable treasure trove of insights into the nature of the human psyche. So convincing is the evidence in favor of past life influences that one can only conclude that those who refuse to consider this to be an area worthy of serious study must either be uninformed or excessively narrow-minded.[122]

Tarthang Tulku, a recognized reincarnated lama of the Nyingmapa lineage of Tibetan Buddhism, wrote in 2002:

> The knowledge of how to control the mind to shape the process of rebirth has been passed on by the great lineage holders of the past. There are works that describe in detail practices for taking rebirth knowingly and how to perfect and refine this capacity of mind through meditation much as a chemist might use chemical reactions possible only under rarified conditions to create a new molecule.[123]

So we seem to have a science of conscious reincarnation as well as new psychological sciences interested in human conception. Meanwhile, changes are leading physical science to a new appreciation of psychic and spiritual phenomena. Because many people, including spiritual teachers and renowned scientists, believe in reincarnation, traditional and current knowledge of that important subject can help us understand the nature of the awareness that may be incarnating at conception.

Reincarnation may be a most important fact of life, and one that may be known directly through inherent human capability. Transpersonal conscious recall of the moment of conception and other early embryonic experiences have in fact been obtained in meditation, in spontaneous recall by young children, in the process of regression therapies, in hypnotherapy, in body psychotherapies, in LSD-assisted psychotherapy, and in various other altered state experiences. In Tibetan Buddhism, conception is the culmination of the "bardo of becoming," the passage from death and thereafter back into life.

My teachers believed in reincarnation, and they seemed to have sensitivity to past lives. But in the lifetimes of my teachers, the earth's population added more than six billion lives. I ask: Where do all these people come from? Given the growth of the human population, we can't reincarnate on a solely individual basis: there must be an inter-connectivity of the collective consciousness, both past and present.

If we all have inherent primal awareness and the collective uncon-scious, we can carry some subtle but powerful traces of the past. Awareness is always free of mind and the past. We may also carry new universal superfields.

Yes, I think it's important to discuss reincarnation at least once in childbirth education courses. The incoming life may be more uni-versal than it's ever been, but it has to work with its ancestry, human language, and unprecedented dangers.

The Nature of Awareness

In contemporary science it's common to use the word "mind" as equiv-alent to "consciousness" or "awareness." From the point of view of meditation science, people must distinguish between mind and aware-ness. Awareness is deep, innate cognition, including intuition. It's an act of knowing, inherently free of mind. Awareness may be an essential characteristic of the universal field and has been referred to as univer-sal mind. It is capable of being cognizant of itself, of its mind, and of external phenomena all at the same time. Human awareness is timeless and formless and may be negentropic, ceaseless and unchanging.

Mind has been more difficult to define. It constantly changes. It's discontinuous. It's intensely concerned with time. It thinks and speaks about itself frequently. It has genetically based qualities and qualities developed after infancy through language and other cultural experi-ences. Some energies of mind may be caused by reincarnation. In the following statements by eminent scientists, the word "mind" is used for what in prenatal meditation we're calling "awareness." Please be patient with that.

Dr. Larry Dossey writes that "Life sciences, such as biology and medicine, are not used to dealing with nonmaterial entities"[124] like mind, but physics is. In the advance of science in the twentieth century, the world enthusiastically received the work of great physicists, including Einstein, Schrödinger, Margenau, and Bohm, who were able to explain mind as a field affecting matter but not caused by it. Dossey comments:

> What has happened is that biologists, who once postulated a privileged role for the human mind in nature's hierarchy, have been moving relentlessly toward the hard-core materialism that characterized nineteenth century physics. At the same time, physicists, faced with compelling experimental evidence, have been moving away from strictly mechanical models of the universe to a view that sees the mind as playing an integral role in all physical events.[125]

In contrast to a biologist or medical researcher who still insists that mind is a product of brain function, Dr. Margenau observes:

> The nonmaterial mind [with the properties of a field] may be completely free and independent from the physical brain, yet fully capable of influencing it, without having to furnish any of the energy required in the transaction between the two. In very complicated physical systems such as the brain, the neurons and sense organs, whose constituents are small enough to be governed by probabilistic quantum laws, the physical organ is always poised for a multitude of possible changes, each with a definite probability; if one change takes place that requires energy … the intricate organism furnishes it automatically. Hence, even if the mind has anything to do with the change, that is, if there is a mind-body interaction, the mind would not be called on to furnish energy.[126]

But where does the mind come from, if not from the brain? To the Nobel Prize laureate physicist Erwin Schrödinger, mind is universal and immortal. Any individual mind is the universal mind. Mind is one mind, transpersonal, timeless, and nonlocal. Replace Schrödinger's word "mind" with "awareness" and it works better, but in either case he was speaking of our universal nature.

Nobel Prize laureates Einstein, Gödel, and Bohm all agree that "Deep down the consciousness of all mankind is one; and if we don't see this it's because we're blinding ourselves to it."[127] The agreement of these eminent scientists is that not only is there a unification of awareness in its universal nature, but it is also, in its essential non-locality, timeless.

The freedom of inherent awareness is a healthful resource for people responding to the intense demands of human time and space, the life we're born into. Mind is chaotic, ego-centered thought, anxiously involved with time. Awareness provides a basis for the experience of timeless freedom.

Sensitivity to the cognitive potential of what incarnates can be the basis of increased respect for the prenatal process, respect that can be cultivated through new educational norms.

The Need for Healthy Childbirth Options

On the World Wide Web, you can see that some people, via the United Nations and elsewhere, are trying to legally define women's and infants' rights in childbirth as a basis of a turnaround in childbirth health care. It's a legal and educational problem.

Today very few pregnant women in America attend any kind of childbirth education class, and the majority of those people go to free classes in hospitals that tend to set them up for medical interventions. Most women gather information from the web and from friends and family while America's tragic birth health statistics call out for widespread health-oriented childbirth education.

Today women sometimes confess to feeling humiliated or cheated out of a normal birth experience after being routinely subjected to a series of medical interventions, depriving the women of personal power. In those many cases, the interventions may be depressing and detrimental for the woman's psychological and physiological health and may adversely impact her child's body and mind. Due to cultural norms and inclinations, many women, particularly because of fear of pain, would choose medicated birth without hesitation. All such women need help. They need to learn that they have noninvasive childbirth options.

Though advances in medicine can be very helpful in problematic births, about one out of ten, the World Health Organization continues to warn that the medications commonly used in childbirth are often unproven as to their safety and carry serious risks, hence the many malpractice lawsuits. Some of the drugs that have been used are known to be toxic. Because the infant's liver is not yet fully developed, she or he is particularly vulnerable. Clearly, medicated birth has serious risks, but women routinely consent to the medical procedures without being adequately informed about the risks. Pregnant women need crucial childbirth education.

For illuminating the variety of traumas caused by unaware professionals and parents in the prevalent way of birth, we can thank contributors to the *Journal of Prenatal and Perinatal Psychology and Health*, from 1986 to the present. Practitioners in this new field are developing therapies to resolve primal wounds from childbirth. For a broad and knowledgeable assessment of birth around the world, we can thank Dr. Marsden Wagner. His work for the World Health Organization has helped expose the tragic risks that come with unnatural childbirth.

Some educators believe that drugs tend to remove the woman's attention from each contraction, which would be focusing exactly on the child in its descent, causing psychic abandonment of the child caught in the muscular contractions. In contrast, focused and uninterrupted caring attention by the woman on her child during labor and delivery may be sustained by the use of deep breathing meditation, allowing the child uninterrupted rapport with the mother during the birth. For the health of our society, we urgently need undisturbed birth.

Perhaps no one has written about the crisis of women in childbirth more meaningfully than Sarah Buckley, MD, an Australian family physician who delivered her own four children at home, including an unattended breech delivery. "Just as we are now discovering the comprehensive benefits of breastfeeding, so we may, in the coming years, come to appreciate the biological intricacy, and the evolutionary wisdom, of normal birth."[128]

New childbirth options, including mind-body medicine, are available and really can help women have wisdom and integrity in childbirth. There is a vital need to educate women about how empowering and healthful birth can be.

Pregnant women who may be headed toward a medical birth,
please prepare with prenatal meditation. It empowers your
immune system and your child's to help you both manage the
side effects of medical birth, and it helps the women heal faster
from any surgeries that may be involved.

Pregnant women who want to have a natural childbirth,
please prepare with prenatal meditation. It can be empowering
for you and the child.

Methods that may be vital for childbirth are available to women from traditional sources and from mind-body medicine. We have methods worthy of respect that can give women profound and healing self-respect. Mind-body self-care practices can help women emerge as protectors of the human potential.

It's clear that if partners do the practices with the pregnant women, for optimal fetal enhancement, for many partners as well as for the women preparing to give birth, it is an opportunity to transform. When partners come together to practice methods to raise the quality of the childbirth and the quality of their lives, childbirth has become a saving grace.

Now, in the twenty-first century, women are able to give birth with more knowledge and probably greater intention than ever before. Childbirth education needs to show women that they have options to birth in a greater way. Let's end this book with the intention that women increasingly give birth in a greater way. May we birth in a greater way.

Glossary

Advanced natural childbirth: New childbirth methods in which meditation practices give women empowering means to adhere to and advance the principles of natural childbirth.

Ancient wisdom methods: Various self-development and healing methods from traditional meditation science, proved through ages of use and currently increasingly appreciated by Western science.

Audioguidance: The use of advanced audio technology to guide those who listen to shift into greater function; an advanced basis of discipline.

Biophoton (from the Greek *bios* meaning "life" and *phos* meaning "light"): A photon of nonthermal origin in the visible and ultraviolet spectrum emitted from a biological system.

Chi **[*Qi*]:** Vital energy. There is external and internal chi. "Chi is fundamental to Chinese medical thinking, yet no one English word or phrase can adequately capture its meaning. Perhaps we can think of *chi* as matter on the verge of becoming energy or energy at the point of materializing."*

Childbirth meditation: The practice of meditation in prenatal care as a means of enrichment, and in postnatal care as a valuable self-care method. The methods may be from any one of a number of available traditions of meditation science.

Complementary and alternative medicine (CAM): The term for various medical disciplines, mostly traditional, now included in the expanded medical paradigm. Dissatisfaction with conventional medical practices has created great popular interest in and respect for CAM.

Complete breathing: Deep breathing of oxygen and vital energy simultaneously; breathing into the physical body and the energy body at the same time.

---

* Kaptchuk, *The Web That Has No Weaver*, 35.

Energy body: The inner body or subtle body of energy channels, energy power centers (chakras), and the subtle but powerful life-giving energy that runs in the energy body channels (chi, prana). Recognized by the National Institutes of Health in 1986.

Energy medicine: Medical practices in which the body is seen to be a body of energy systems and fields; practices of seeing and modifying those fields therapeutically constitute diagnosis and treatment. Acupuncture, acupressure, bodywork, and conscious breathing are each a kind of energy medicine.

Enriched pregnancy: Childbirth practices, including playing good music, reading to the wombchild, and meditation, used in prenatal care to access the optimal health and developmental potential in childbirth.

Expanded anatomy: The systems of human multidimensional anatomy, the inseparable physical body and energy body, offer a vision of what the body is and what functions may be developed through methods of meditation science.

Fine breathing: Deep breathing that intentionally absorbs vital energy from the air as well as accessing optimal oxygenation.

Giving and Receiving: An advanced natural childbirth method that brings the experience of healing into childbirth. It is valuable in both prenatal and postnatal care.

Hara: The vital center; focal point of Zen meditation, comparable to and perhaps the same as the *tan tien* in Chinese T'ai Chi meditation and the Life Vase (*bum chung*) in Tibetan Vajrayana meditation. It is a receiver for energies breathed into it, for greater function and increase of life force.

Meditation: A consciousness discipline that enables people to experience greater levels of awareness and health, normally blocked by the mind in its undisciplined activity.

Meditation science: The scientific knowledge behind meditation methods from different traditions, with understanding of the short- and long-term effects of the application of those methods. These methods have been tested and proved through centuries of disciplined use, yielding repeatable results.

Mind-body medicine: An important development in the history of medicine, expanding the medical paradigm in the West since the 1970s, in which meditation and other interventions using the mind enable the body to improve its function. Called self-care, it's seen as the heart of a new medical paradigm.

Mindfulness-Based Stress Reduction: The renowned mind-body medicine clinic at the University of Massachusetts Medical Center. Established in 1979, it has trained more than twenty thousand people in medicine/meditation methods and has been the model for hundreds of such programs established in America, Canada, and Europe.

Negentrophy (Negentropic): Entrophy implies a living system that increases in complexity tending to break down and lose potential. Negentrophy is a force in living systems that restores order and potential. This is probably caused by the vast amount of free energy available everywhere anytime (zero-point energy).

Optimal childbirth breathing: Breathing practice, such as Womb Breathing, in which vital energy from the air as well as full oxygenation are breathed, enriching the child with energy and developmental intention.

Paradigm: A pattern, example, or model. A concept accepted by most people in an intellectual community, as those in one of the natural sciences, because it seems to be effective in explaining a complex process, idea, or set of data.

Paradigm shift: A change in the way individuals or cultures see the world, or interpret phenomena, giving people a sense of having new eyes or new knowing. Paradigm shifts are caused by evolutionary progress, setting people free of restrictive conditioning.

Placenta: The soft, spongy organ through which the woman's blood nourishes the fetus, through the umbilical cord; it is expelled after birth, sometimes treated as sacred and buried as such. In optimal birth, the umbilical cord is not cut as long as it is pulsing oxygen and nourishment to the child, which could be for an hour or more.

Practice of Opening: An advanced natural childbirth method using a reclining progressive relaxation technique. Those who do the practice are brought into life force in their cellular nature in various ways, resulting in nervous system healing, increased knowledge of the body and its capabilities, and direct developmental connection with the wombchild.

Prana: A subtle but powerful life energy pervading all matter; universal life force. Probably the same as chi. Current science refers to it as universal energy and speaks of its field being measurable. It can be breathed and utilized, as in the practice of Womb Breathing.

Shamatha (Sanskrit): Calm abiding. A meditation practice for calming down and staying calm in order to rest free of the disturbances of the mind. Various concentration techniques are used. The most common is following the breath.

Slow breathing: Deep, abdominal breathing becomes slow breathing, healthier breathing using minimal energy. Ancient wisdom says that each life has a certain amount of breaths to live, and intentionally slow breathing brings long life.

Subtle body: Inner body, or energy body. Traditionally, esoteric systems envisioned several bodies inherent in the physical body. Sometimes called astral, mental, and causal bodies, these bodies have been seen to be operating at successively higher frequencies than the physical body. They are engaged, activated, and utilized by evolutionary work. Medicine today accepts the presence of an energy body in the physical body, in which subtle body functions are integral to physical functions.

Sympathetic resonance: Sympathetic resonance or sympathetic vibration is a harmonic phenomenon wherein a formerly passive string or vibratory body responds to external vibrations to which it has a harmonic likeness.

Tan tien: Focal point for T'ai Chi meditation, situated in the navel center. The tan tien is similar to the Life Vase and the hara, and may be the same.

Umbilicus: The depression in the center of the abdomen where the umbilical cord has been cut; the navel.

Vajrayana: The Diamond Vehicle; the Buddhism of Tibet; the ultimate stage of the development of the Buddha's teachings. Based on the vow of compassionate service to all life, Vajrayana Buddhism is known for its variety of profound methods.

Vase breathing: This practice, a treasure of ancient wisdom, is characterized by breathing vital essence in the air down into the Life Vase, *bum chung* (in Tibetan), in the navel center, which feeds the energy up into the central psychic channel for greater function.

Vipashyana (Sanskrit): Clear or wider seeing; panoramic awareness; extraordinary insight; "Wisdom Mind" arising from Shamatha practice.

Visualization: Most often a concentration method in which the whole body, a specific body system, or a body process is envisioned purposefully, to alter the body's biology beneficially. To be most successful, visualization should be based on calming meditation.

Wise Woman tradition: The ancient understanding that in every community there were women who held and shared the wisdom of previous generations for the well-being of all. They were healers, teachers, midwives, and coordinators of community-wide events and ceremonies. They participated with other elders in decision making for the community. Historically in indigenous Western culture a Wise Woman was in charge of the main temple. She married the king and co-ruled with him.

Womb Breathing: A method of advanced natural childbirth developed from traditional meditation science. Using a new vision of the body of the pregnant woman, extending childbirth anatomy, this deep breathing practice gives women an expanded sense of their natural birthing capabilities.

World Health Organization: The international health and research services of the United Nations.

Yoga: Literally "union." Originally a general category for various kinds of meditation practice, today in the West, yoga usually refers to hatha yoga, stretching and breathing exercises, which can be beneficial in prenatal care.

Zygote: The union of male and female reproductive cells that develops into a new individual.

Resources

About Calm Birth

Calm Birth is an international childbirth program that trains pregnant women and childbirth professionals in a new childbirth practice.

Though Calm Birth originated in American hospitals, primarily in Oregon, California, and New Jersey, from 1997 onward, Calm Birth has been developing teacher training programs in England and Australia, and elsewhere around the globe.

Calm Birth is both a new childbirth practice and a new kind of childbirth education. It is endorsed by leading childbirth educators, including Christiane Northrup, MD: "Calm Birth is a sublime gift to all of us ... The positive impact of Calm Birth on society can't be overestimated."

CalmBirth.org will connect you to the programs and teachers of this childbirth practice.

Christine Novak of Calm Birth was awarded the March of Dimes Best for Baby award in 2009 for bringing Calm Birth into the New Jersey hospital system.

Calm Birth offers both prenatal and postnatal practices for women to learn to function more completely, with complete breathing and meditation.

The complete breathing of Calm Birth helps women shift into greater function, for self-development and for prenatal child development.

For information about Calm Birth services and products, please visit: www.calmbirth.org.

References

Achterberg, Jeanne. *Imagery in Healing: Shamanism and Modern Medicine.* Boston: Shambhala, 1985.

Achterberg, Jeanne. *Woman as Healer.* Boston: Shambhala, 1990.

Astin, John. "Stress Reduction through Mindfulness Meditation: Effects on Psychological Symptomatology, Sense of Control, and Spiritual Experiences." *Psychotherapy and Psychosomatics* 66 (1997): 97–106.

Baker, Jeannine Parvati. *Prenatal Yoga and Natural Childbirth.* Berkeley, CA: North Atlantic Books, 1974.

Bardsley, Sandra. *Creating a Joyful Birth Experience: Developing a Partnership with Your Unborn Child for Healthy Pregnancy, Labor, and Early Parenting* (New York: Simon & Schuster, 1994).

Benson, Herbert. *Timeless Healing: The Power and Biology of Belief.* New York: Simon & Schuster, 1996.

Bohm, David. *Wholeness and the Implicate Order.* London: Routledge, 1980.

Borysenko, Joan, and Miroslav Borysenko. *The Power of the Mind to Heal.* Carson, CA: Hay House, 1994.

Bradley, Robert. *Husband-Coached Childbirth.* New York: Harper & Row, 1974.

Braid, James. *Neurypnology or the Rationale of Nervous Sleep.* London: J. Churchill, 1846.

Brennan, Barbara. *Hands of Light.* New York: Bantam Books, 1988.

_____. *Light Emerging.* New York: Bantam Books, 1993.

Buckley, Sarah. *Gentle Birth, Gentle Mothering.* Berkeley, CA: Celestial Arts, 2005.

Cardoso, Roberto, et al. "Meditation in Health: An Operational Definition." *Brain Research Protocols* 14 (2004), www.elsevier.com.

Castaneda, Carlos. *A Separate Reality.* New York: Pocket Books, 1971.

_____. *Magical Passes.* New York: HarperCollins, 1998.

Chamberlain, David. *The Mind of Your Newborn Baby.* Berkeley, CA: North Atlantic Books, 1998.

_____. "Selected Works by David Chamberlain." *Journal of Prenatal and Perinatal Psychology and Health* 14, nos. 1–2 (1999): 1–194.

_____. *Windows to the Womb: Revealing the Conscious Baby from Conception to Birth*. Berkeley, CA: North Atlantic Books, 2013.

Chan, Ka Po. "Effects of Perinatal Meditation on Pregnant Chinese Women in Hong Kong: A Randomized Controlled Trial." *Journal of Nursing Education and Practice* 5, no. 1 (2014): 1–18.

Chang, Garma C. C. *The Six Yogas of Naropa*. Ithaca, NY: Snow Lion, 1963.

Ch'ing, Cheng Man. *Cheng Tzu's Thirteen Treatises on T'ai Chi Ch'uan*. Berkeley, CA: North Atlantic Books, 1985.

Chopra, Deepak. *Quantum Healing: Exploring the Frontiers of Mind-Body Medicine*. New York: Bantam Books, 1990.

Davis-Floyd, Robbie. *Birth as an American Rite of Passage*. Berkeley: University of California Press, 2003.

Dick-Read, Grantly. *Childbirth without Fear*. New York: Harper & Row, 1944.

Dossey, Larry. *Recovering the Soul*. New York: Bantam, 1989.

_____. *Healing Words: The Power of Prayer and the Practice of Medicine*. New York: HarperOne, 1995.

_____. *Reinventing Medicine*. San Francisco: HarperOne, 1998.

Einstein, Albert. *Ideas and Opinions*. New York: Crown, 1954.

Ferguson, Marilyn. *The Aquarian Conspiracy*. Los Angeles: J. P. Tarcher, 1980.

Gaskin, Ina May. *Ina May's Guide to Childbirth*. New York: Bantam/Dell, 2003.

Gauld, Alan. *A History of Hypnotism*. New York: Cambridge University Press, 1992.

Goleman, Daniel, and Joel Gurin, eds. *Mind-Body Medicine*. Yonkers, NY: Consumer Reports Books, 1993.

Grof, Stanislav. *The Holotropic Mind: The Three Levels of Consciousness and How They Shape Our Lives*. New York: HarperCollins, 1993.

Hallett, Elisabeth. *Soul Trek: Meeting Our Children on the Way to Birth*. Hamilton, MT: Light Hearts, 1995.

Harding, John H., and John V. Timko. "The Use of Psychotropic Medications during Pregnancy and Lactation." *Global Library of Women's Medicine*, 2008.

Hayward, Jeremy, and Karen Hayward. *Sacred World*. Boston: Shambhala, 2001.

Hendricks, Gay. *Conscious Breathing: Breathwork for Health, Stress Release, and Personal Mastery*. New York: Simon & Schuster, 1995.

Hooper, Judith. "Ommm … Please Pass the DHEA." *Health* 21 (1989): 34.

Huch, Renate. "Maternal Hyperventilation and the Fetus." *Journal of Prenatal Medicine* 14, no. 3 (1986): 3–17.

Hughes, Annie, et al. "Mindfulness Approaches to Childbirth and Parenting." *British Journal of Midwifery* 17, no. 10 (2009): 630–635.

Jacobson, Edmund. *Progressive Relaxation.* Chicago: University of Chicago Press, 1938.

James, William. *Varieties of Religious Experience.* New York: Collier, 1961.

Journal of Prenatal and Perinatal Psychology and Health. Forestville, CA: APPPAH, 1986.

Kabat-Zinn, Jon. *Full Catastrophe Living: Using the Wisdom of Your Body and Mind to Face Stress, Pain, and Illness.* New York: Bantam Doubleday Dell, 1990.

Kabat-Zinn, Jon, et al. "Meditation, Melatonin and Breast/Prostate Cancer." *Medical Hypotheses* 44 (1995): 39–46.

Kaptchuk, Ted J. *The Web That Has No Weaver.* New York: Congdon and Weed, 1983.

Khalsa, Dharma Singh, and Cameron Stauth. *Meditation as Medicine.* New York: Simon & Schuster, 2001.

Koren, Gideon, Anne Pastuszak, and Shinya Ito. "Drugs in Pregnancy." *New England Journal of Medicine* 338 (1998): 1128–1137.

Lamaze, Fernand. *Painless Childbirth: The Lamaze Method.* New York: Simon & Schuster, 1965.

Leboyer, Frédérick. *Inner Beauty, Inner Light: Yoga for Pregnant Women.* New York: William Morrow Paperbacks, 1978.

———. *Birth without Violence.* Rochester, NY: Healing Arts Press, 1995.

Margenau, Henry. *The Miracle of Existence.* Boston: New Science Library, 1987.

Michaels, Paula A. "Childbirth Pain Relief and the Soviet Origins of the Lamaze Method." Seattle: NCEEER, 2007.

Montagu, Ashley. *The Natural Superiority of Women.* New York: Macmillan, 1954.

Murphy, Michael, and Steven Donovan. *The Physical and Psychological Effects of Meditation: A Review of Contemporary Research with a Comprehensive Bibliography.* Sausalito, CA: Institute of Noetic Sciences, 1999.

Murphy, Michael, and George Leonard. *The Life We Are Given.* New York: Tarcher/Putnam, 2005.

Myss, Caroline. *Anatomy of the Spirit.* New York: Harmony, 1996.

Myss, Caroline, and Norman Shealy. *The Creation of Health.* Walpole, NH: Stillpoint, 1993.

Newman, Robert Bruce. *Calm Birth: New Method for Conscious Childbirth.* Berkeley, CA: North Atlantic Books, 2005.

Odent, Michel. *Birth Reborn.* Medford, NJ: Birthworks Press, 1994.

Ornish, Dean. *Dr. Dean Ornish's Program for Reversing Heart Disease.* New York: Random House, 1990.

Oschman, James. *Energy Medicine.* Edinburgh, Scotland: Harcourt, 2000.

Oz, Mehmet. *Healing from the Heart.* New York: Penguin Putnam, 1998.

Pelletier, Kenneth R. *Mind as Slayer, Mind as Healer.* New York: Dell, 1977.

Pert, Candace. *Molecules of Emotion.* New York: Simon & Schuster, 1997.

Pierpaoli, Walter, and William Regelson. *The Melatonin Miracle.* New York: Simon & Schuster, 1995.

Rama, Swami, Rudolph Ballentine, and Alan Hymes. *Science of Breath.* Honesdale, PA: Himalayan International Institute of Yogic Science and Philosophy, 1979.

Reilly, Sharon. "The Health Benefits of Meditation for Pregnancy and Birth," The Preventive Medicine Center, www.thepmc.org/category/library/re-sourcesguest-article.

Reiter, Russel J., and Jo Robinson. *Melatonin: Your Body's Natural Wonder Drug.* New York: Bantam Books, 1995.

Rinpoche, Sogyal. *The Tibetan Book of Living and Dying.* San Francisco: HarperSanFrancisco, 1994.

Rosen, Steven. *The Reincarnation Controversy: Uncovering the Truth in the World Religions.* Badger, CA: Torchlight, 1997.

Schlitz, Marilyn, and Tina Amorok. *Consciousness and Healing: Integral Approaches to Mind-Body Medicine.* St. Louis, MO: Churchill Livingston, 2004.

Schrödinger, Erwin. *What Is Life? and Mind and Matter.* London: Cambridge University Press, 1969.

Schwartz, Fred. "Perinatal Stress Reduction, Music and Medical Cost Savings," *Journal of Prenatal and Perinatal Psychology and Health* 12, no. 1 (1997): 1–44.

Sharma, Renu, and Bhupendra M. Palan, eds. *Hypnosis: Psycho-Philosophical Perspectives and Therapeutic Relevance.* New Delhi: Concept, 2011.

Sloan, Frank A., Kathryn Whetten-Goldstein, Penny B. Githens, and Stephen S. Entman. "Effects of the Threat of Medical Malpractice Litigation and Other Factors on Birth Outcomes." *Medical Care* 33, no. 7 (1995): 700–714.

Squier, Raymond. "Integral Medicine: A New Term." *British Journal of Medical Psychology* 19 (1945): 367.

Sriboonpimsuay, Wanlapa, et al. "Meditation for Preterm Birth Prevention: A Randomized Controlled Trial in Udonthani, Thailand." *International Journal of Public Health Research* 1, no. 1 (2011): 31–39.

Swanson, Claude. *Life Force, the Scientific Basis: Volume 2 of the Synchronized Universe Series.* Tucson, AZ: Poseidia Press, 2011.

Tolle, Eckhart. *The Power of Now.* Novato, CA: New World Library, 1999.

Tsai, Sing-Ling, and Mary S. Crockett. "Effects of Relaxation Training, Combining Imagery, and Meditation on the Stress Level of Chinese Nurses Working in Modern Hospitals in Taiwan." *Issues in Mental Health Nursing* 14, no. 1 (1993): 51–66.

Tulku, Tarthang. *Mind over Matter: Reflections on Buddhism in the West.* Berkeley, CA: Dharma, 2002.

Ulin, Priscilla R. *Changing Techniques in Psychoprophylactic Preparation for Childbirth.* New York: Wolters Kluwer Health, 1968.

Verny, Thomas. *The Secret Life of the Unborn Child.* New York: Dell, 1981.

_____. *Tomorrow's Baby: The Art and Science of Parenting from Conception through Infancy.* New York: Simon & Schuster, 2002.

Vieten, Cassandra. *Mindful Motherhood.* Oakland, CA: Noetic Books, New Harbinger, 2009.

Vieten, Cassandra, and John Astin. "Effects of a Mindfulness-Based Intervention during Pregnancy on Prenatal Stress and Mood: Results of a Pilot Study." *Archives of Women's Mental Health* 11, no. 1 (2008): 67–74.

Vivekananda Yoga Research Foundation. "Meditation Benefits for Pregnancy," 2009, cited on www.ecoinstitute.org.

Von Dürckheim, Karlfried G. *Hara.* London: George Allen & Unwin, 1977.

Wagner, Marsden. *The Birth Machine: The Search for Appropriate Birth Technology.* Camperdown, Australia: ACE Graphics, 1994.

Weaver, Judyth. "Encounters with Grandmaster Cheng Man-Ch'ing," 2003, http://judythweaver.com/writings/encounters-with-cheng-man-ching/.

Webster's New World College Dictionary, 3rd ed. New York: Macmillan, 1986.

Wilber, Ken. *The Marriage of Sense and Soul.* Boston: Shambhala, 1998.

_____. *Boomeritis.* Boston: Shambhala, 2002.

Wilhelm, Richard. *The Secret of the Golden Flower.* New York: Wehman Bros., 1955.

Zenji, Hakuin. *The Embossed Tea Kettle.* Sydney: George Allen & Unwin, 1963.

Zohar, Danah. *Quantum Self.* New York: William Morrow Paperbacks, 1990.

Notes

Preface

1 Marilyn Ferguson, *The Aquarian Conspiracy* (Los Angeles: J. P. Tarcher, 1980), 30.

2 Sy Mukherjee, "Giving Birth in the U.S. Costs More Than Anywhere Else in the World," Think Progress, July 1, 2013.

3 Megan Brockett, "Medical Officials Call for Birth Injury Fund to Combat High-Cost Malpractice Lawsuits," Capital News Service, March 11, 2014.

4 Marsden Wagner, "Technology in Birth: First Do No Harm," www.mid -wiferytoday.com/articles/technologyinbirth.htm.

5 Ina May Gaskin, "Maternal Death in the United States," 2008, www.ncbi .nlm.nih.gov.

6 "New Studies Confirm Safety of Home Birth in the United States," Midwives Alliance, January 30, 2014.

I Background

7 Jeanne Achterberg, *Woman as Healer* (Boston: Shambhala, 1990), 198.

8 _____, *Imagery in Healing: Shamanism and Modern Medicine* (Boston: Shambhala, 1985), 67.

9 Achterberg, *Woman as Healer*, 88.

10 Ibid., 81.

11 Ibid., 83.

II Prenatal Meditation

12 Joan Borysenko and Miroslav Borysenko, *The Power of the Mind to Heal* (Carson, CA: Hay House, 1994), 116.

13 Roberto Cardoso et al., "Meditation in Health: An Operational Definition," *Brain Research Protocols* 14 (2004): 58–60.

14 Michael Murphy and Steven Donovan, *The Physical and Psychological Effects of Meditation: A Review of Contemporary Research with a Comprehensive Bibliography* (Sausalito, CA: Institute of Noetic Sciences, 1999), 1.

15 Gideon Koren, Anne Pastuszak, and Shinya Ito, "Drugs in Pregnancy," *New England Journal of Medicine* 338 (1998): 1128–1137.

16 Frank Sloan, Kathryn Whetten-Goldstein, Penny B. Githens, and Stephen S. Entman, "Effects of the Threat of Medical Malpractice Litigation and Other Factors on Birth Outcomes," *Medical Care* 33, no. 7 (1995): 700–714.

17 Ibid.

18 John H. Harding and John V. Timko, "The Use of Psychotropic Medications during Pregnancy and Lactation," *Global Library of Women's Medicine*, 2008.

19 Russel J. Reiter and Jo Robinson, *Melatonin: Your Body's Natural Wonder Drug* (New York: Bantam Books, 1995), 151.

20 Ibid., 71.

21 Deepak Chopra, *Quantum Healing: Exploring the Frontiers of Mind-Body Medicine* (New York: Bantam Books, 1990), 61–62.

22 Michel Odent, *Birth Reborn* (Medford, NJ: Birthworks Press, 1994), 42.

23 Candace Pert, *Molecules of Emotion* (New York: Simon & Schuster, 1997), 186.

24 Murphy and Donovan. *The Physical and Psychological Effects of Meditation,* 81–87.

25 Ibid.

26 Cassandra Vieten and John Astin, "Effects of a Mindfulness-Based Intervention during Pregnancy on Prenatal Stress and Mood: Results of a Pilot Study," *Archives of Women's Mental Health* 11, no. 1 (2008): 67–74.

27 Annie Hughes et al. "Mindfulness Approaches to Childbirth and Parenting," *British Journal of Midwifery* 17, no. 10 (2009): 630–635.

28 Vivekananda Yoga Research Foundation, "Meditation Benefits for Pregnancy," 2009, cited on www.ecoinstitute.org.

29 Wanlapa Sriboonpimsuay et al., "Meditation for Preterm Birth Prevention: A Randomized Controlled Trial in Udonthani, Thailand," *International Journal of Public Health Research* 1, no. 1 (2011): 31–39.

30 Ibid.

31 Ka Po Chan, "Effects of Perinatal Meditation on Pregnant Chinese Women in Hong Kong: A Randomized Controlled Trial," *Journal of Nursing Education and Practice* 5, no. 1 (2014): 1–18.

32 John Astin, "Stress Reduction through Mindfulness Meditation: Effects on Psychological Symptomatology, Sense of Control, and Spiritual Experiences," *Psychotherapy and Psychosomatics* 66 (1997): 97–106.

33 Murphy and Donovan, *The Physical and Psychological Effects of Meditation,* 81–87.

34 Robbie Davis-Floyd. *Birth as an American Rite of Passage* (Berkeley: University of California Press, 2003), 99.

III Childbirth in the Human Energy System

35 Caroline Myss, *Anatomy of the Spirit* (New York: Harmony, 1996), 33.

36 Barbara Brennan, *Hands of Light* (New York: Bantam Books, 1988), 21.

37 James Oschman, *Energy Medicine* (Edinburgh, Scotland: Harcourt, 2000), 145.

38 Claude Swanson, *Life Force, the Scientific Basis: Volume 2 of the Synchronized Universe Series* (Tucson, AZ: Poseidia Press, 2011).

39 Oschman, *Energy Medicine*, 145.

40 Frédérick Leboyer, *Inner Beauty, Inner Light: Yoga for Pregnant Women* (New York: William Morrow Paperbacks, 1978), 142–143.

41 Ibid.

42 Jeannine Parvati Baker, *Prenatal Yoga and Natural Childbirth* (Berkeley, CA: North Atlantic Books, 1974), xii.

43 Ibid., xiii.

44 Ibid., 18.

45 Ibid., 2.

46 Ibid., 77.

47 Ibid., 88.

48 Ibid., 90.

49 Dean Ornish, *Dr. Dean Ornish's Program for Reversing Heart Disease* (New York: Random House, 1990), 165.

IV Pregnancy as a Path of Human Development and Evolution

50 Pert, *Molecules of Emotion*, 186.

51 Carlos Castaneda, *Magical Passes* (New York: HarperCollins, 1998), 71.

52 Ashley Montagu, *The Natural Superiority of Women* (New York: Macmillan, 1954).

53 Cheng Man Ch'ing, *Cheng Tzu's Thirteen Treatises on T'ai Chi Ch'uan* (Berkeley, CA: North Atlantic Books, 1985), 77.

54 Ibid.

55 Judyth Weaver, "Encounters with Grandmaster Cheng Man-Ch'ing," 2003, http://judythweaver.com/writings/encounters-with-cheng-man-ching/.

56 Karlfried G. Von Dürckheim, *Hara* (London: George Allen & Unwin, 1977), 57.

57 Ibid., 107.

58 Ibid., 123.

59 Ibid., 137–138.

60 Ibid., 142.

61 Hakuin Zenji, *The Embossed Tea Kettle* (Sydney: George Allen & Unwin, 1963), 40.

62 Ibid., 31.

63 Ibid., 41.

64 Ibid., 67.

65 Richard Wilhelm, *The Secret of the Golden Flower* (New York: Wehman Bros., 1955), 57.

66 Eckhart Tolle, *The Power of Now* (Novato, CA: New World Library, 1999), 138–141.

67 Ibid., 142.

V The Calm Birth Method

68 Castaneda, *Magical Passes*, 27.

69 Kathleen Michon, "Medical Malpractice: Common Errors by Doctors and Hospitals," www.nolo.com.

70 Kenneth R. Pelletier, *Mind as Slayer, Mind as Healer* (New York: Dell, 1977), 197.

71 Gay Hendricks, *Conscious Breathing: Breathwork for Health, Stress Release, and Personal Mastery* (New York: Simon & Schuster, 1995), 19–20.

72 Jeremy Hayward and Karen Hayward, *Sacred World* (Boston: Shambhala, 2001), 78.

73 Odent, *Birth Reborn*, 13.

VI Calm Births

74 Ina May Gaskin, *Ina May's Guide to Childbirth* (New York: Bantam / Dell, 2003), 4.

VII Calm Mother Practices: Empowering Postnatal Care

75 Davis-Floyd, *Birth as an American Rite of Passage*, 41.

VIII New Childbirth Medicine

76 Stanislav Grof, *The Holotropic Mind: The Three Levels of Consciousness and How They Shape Our Lives* (New York: HarperCollins, 1993), 201.

77 David Chamberlain, *The Mind of Your Newborn Baby* (Berkeley, CA: North Atlantic Books, 1998), 224.

78 Ibid., 22.

79 Fred Schwartz, "Perinatal Stress Reduction, Music and Medical Cost Savings," *Journal of Prenatal and Perinatal Psychology and Health* 12, no. 1 (1997), 27.

80 Danah Zohar, *Quantum Self* (New York: William Morrow Paperbacks, 1990), 141–147.

81 Elisabeth Hallett, *Soul Trek: Meeting Our Children on the Way to Birth* (Hamilton, MT: Light Hearts, 1995), 54.

82 Ken Wilber, *The Marriage of Sense and Soul* (Boston: Shambhala, 1998), 168.

83 Ibid., 170.

84 Ibid., 190.

IX The Evolution of Mind-Body Practice in Obstetrics

85 Marilyn Schlitz and Tina Amorok, *Consciousness and Healing: Integral Approaches to Mind-Body Medicine* (St. Louis, MO: Churchill Livingstone, 2004), xxxiii.

86 Achterberg, *Imagery in Healing*, 90.

87 Mehmet Oz, *Healing from the Heart* (New York: Penguin Putnam, 1998), 16.

88 Renu Sharma and Bhupendra M. Palan, eds., *Hypnosis: Psycho-Philosophical Perspectives and Therapeutic Relevance* (New Delhi: Concept, 2011), 74.

89 American Society of Clinical Hypnosis.

90 Alex Lyda, "Hypnosis Gaining Ground in Medicine," Columbia News.

91 Daniel Goleman and Joel Gurin, eds., *Mind-Body Medicine* (Yonkers, NY: Consumer Reports Books, 1993), 278.

92 Alan Gauld, *A History of Hypnotism* (New York: Cambridge University Press, 1992).

93 James Braid, *Neurypnology or the Rationale of Nervous Sleep* (London: J. Churchill, 1846), 214–216.

94 Ibid.

95 Fernand Lamaze, *Painless Childbirth: The Lamaze Method* (New York: Simon & Schuster, 1965), 22.

96 Ibid., 25.

97 Ibid.

98 Ibid., 32.

99 Ibid., 23.

100 Achterberg, *Imagery in Healing*, 90.

101 Ibid., 28.

102 Odent, *Birth Reborn*, 12.

103 Lamaze, *Painless Childbirth*, 13.

104 Renate Huch, "Maternal Hyperventilation and the Fetus," *Journal of Prenatal Medicine* 14, no. 3 (1986): 3–17.

105 Murphy and Donovan, *The Physical and Psychological Effects of Meditation*, 51.

106 Cassandra Vieten, *Mindful Motherhood* (Oakland, CA: Noetic Books, New Harbinger, 2009).

107 Robert Bruce Newman, *Calm Birth: New Method for Conscious Childbirth* (Berkeley, CA: North Atlantic Books, 2005), 69.

108 Ibid., 56.

109 Ibid., 42.

110 Achterberg, *Imagery in Healing*, 186.

111 Schlitz and Amorok, *Consciousness and Healing*, xv.

X Toward a New Era of Childbirth Education

112 Caroline Myss and Norman Shealy, *The Creation of Health* (Walpole, NH: Stillpoint, 1993), 126.

113 Michael Murphy and George Leonard, *The Life We Are Given* (New York: Tarcher/Putnam, 2005), 172.

114 Ferguson, *The Aquarian Conspiracy*, 74.

115 Odent, *Birth Reborn*, 35.

116 Larry Dossey, *Healing Words: The Power of Prayer and the Practice of Medicine* (New York: HarperOne, 1995), 18.

117 David Chamberlain, *Windows to the Womb: Revealing the Conscious Baby from Conception to Birth* (Berkeley, CA: North Atlantic Books, 2013).

118 Thomas Verny, *The Secret Life of the Unborn Child* (New York: Dell, 1981); Thomas Verny, *Tomorrow's Baby: The Art and Science of Parenting from Conception through Infancy* (New York: Simon & Schuster, 2002).

119 Chamberlain, "Selected Works by David Chamberlain," *Journal of Prenatal and Perinatal Psychology and Health*, 4/98, 86–87.

120 Chamberlain, *Windows to the Womb*, 175.

121 Ibid.

122 Grof, *The Holotropic Mind*, 126–127.

123 Tarthang Tulku, *Mind over Matter: Reflections on Buddhism in the West* (Berkeley, CA: Dharma, 2002), 43.

124 Larry Dossey, *Recovering the Soul* (New York: Bantam, 1989), 175.

125 Ibid., 176.

126 Henry Margenau, *The Miracle of Existence* (Boston: New Science Library, 1987), 165.

127 Dossey, *Recovering the Soul*, 78.

128 Sarah Buckley, *Gentle Birth, Gentle Mothering* (Berkeley, CA: Celestial Arts, 2005), 69.

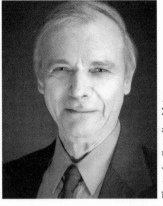

About the Author

When he was young, ROBERT BRUCE NEWMAN wanted to be a doctor. He enrolled in college and studied in a pre-med program. After three years, he switched majors and received a BA degree in English literature from the University of California at Berkeley. It was after college that his real studies began. In 1967 he began to work with teachers trained in profound methods from meditation science traditions. In 1970 he began a ten-year study and practice of Shamatha Vipashyana meditation with Chögyam Trungpa Rinpoche, a Tibetan Vajrayana Buddhist meditation teacher. This practice is essentially the same as the one used in the University of Massachusetts Medical Center's medicine/meditation program. From 1980 to the present Mr. Newman has been working with Vajrayana meditation teachers who are also doctors. He was trained for many years in a deep breathing method called vase breathing, breathing vital energy, which became the basis of his work in the medical uses of meditation.

Though he has taught various courses in colleges and universities—including the University of Colorado at Boulder, the City University of New York, and Naropa University—Mr. Newman's teaching of meditation remained private until 1991, the same year the National Institutes of Health established its National Center for Complementary and Alternative Medicine. It was then, with Dr. John Sutton and Dr. Craig Spaniol of NASA, and Dr. Ted Wolff of NYU Medical Center, that MediGrace, Inc., was incorporated for the research and development of medical and childbirth uses of meditation.

The first MediGrace program was a medicine/meditation program using three practices: Practice of Deep Release; Vase Breathing; and Empathic Healing. From 1997 to 2004, more than sixty Medical Uses of Meditation trainings were presented in West Coast hospitals, with education credits via the California Board of Registered Nursing.

The second program that evolved was Calm Birth. Mr. Newman has been president of MediGrace since 1991, and a Calm Birth teacher trainer since 1997.

In 2005, this book Newman's first book on childbirth meditation was published for the first time: *Calm Birth: New Method for Conscious Childbirth*. In 2006 his first book on the use of meditation in medicine was published, with Ruth L. Miller: *Calm Healing: Methods for a New Era of Medicine*.

ALSO BY ROBERT BRUCE NEWMAN

available from North Atlantic Books

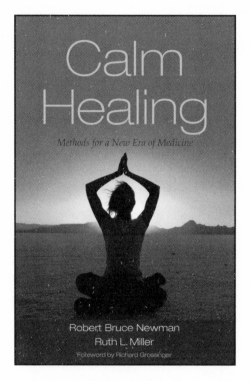

Calm Healing

978-1-55643-626-0 (print)
978-1-62317-058-5 (ebook)

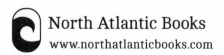

North Atlantic Books
www.northatlanticbooks.com

North Atlantic Books is an independent, nonprofit publisher committed to a bold exploration of the relationships between mind, body, spirit, and nature.